# Essential Oils

*(Aromatherapy 101)*

*Tackling Stress Relief, Enhancing Life, Beauty, Youth, Energy via Essential Oils*

# Table of Contents

# Introduction

It has long been understood by scientists that scents have a very specific role to play when it comes to the human brain.

Scents may warn us that something is not good to eat, that there is danger ahead, or a familiar childhood scent can stimulate the memory center of the brain and help us take our minds back to happy moments.

Considering the impact of smell on our minds, it is therefore not surprising that scents can be used to promote healing and calm as well.

And so, enter stage left, Aromatherapy. Mirriam Webster's Dictionary defines "aromatherapy" as, "the use of natural oils that have a pleasant smell to make a person feel better especially by rubbing the oils into the skin."

Aromatherapy makes use of essential oils derived from plants in order to produce healing effects on body and mind. This form of treatment is completely natural and, as long as the guidelines are followed, entirely safe.

Some of the essential oils are even gentle enough to be used during pregnancy or on your baby.

Oils can thus be incorporated at most stages of life, improving not only your health and well-being, but that of your family as well.

In this book I will go through the basics of aromatherapy - which oils to choose, how to blend and use them and safety precautions that should be followed at all times.

Having read through this book, you will be equipped with enough information to allow you to make your own aromatherapy oils and blends to successfully treat minor ailments that may crop up, create your own personal cosmetics and scent and help to freshen your home.

Essential oils do more than just smell good - they are potent healers and great antibacterial agents as well.

Start your journey today and you will feel like a new person in no time flat. Regain your energy, finally beat stress and look and feel your best and then help your family to do the same - even your family dog can benefit from the proper use of essential oils.

This book is crammed with information and I am sure that you will learn a lot. Once you have read through the basics and understand how to work with essential oils safely, you can pick and choose sections according to what interests you. Whether you want a magic potion to make you look younger or just need a quick energy boost, you'll find help here.

# Chapter 1: Why Use Aromatherapy?

## Your Journey to Health and Happiness Begins Now

Most of us are familiar with aromatherapy in one way or another. Even if you have not specifically gone for an aromatherapy treatment, you are bound to have bought a product that contained essential oils at one stage or another.

Aromatherapy is not some new age hippy-dippy treatment - it has been around for thousands of years and is even used today in medical centers around the globe to help reduce the spread of infectious bacteria and to help promote the healing of patients.

Essential oils such as Eucalyptus and Tea Tree oil are particularly prized for their strong anti-bacterial and anti-viral effects. So potent in fact that the oils need only be diffused into the atmosphere in order to get rid of air-borne viruses.

Some oils are used to benefit the body and to fight disease at a physical level. Others act in a more subtle manner to help to heal the mind.

Why use aromatherapy? Essential oils are natural, concentrated healing essences that can be applied in several different ways allowing you to tailor your treatment plan to the one that suits you and the members of your family best.

Each plant essence is made up of different elements, depending on the plant it was derived from and the particular needs that plant had and so different essences can have vastly different properties making them extremely useful and versatile.

Take Sandalwood oil, for example. You can add it to your night cream to help intensely moisturize dry skin; add into your husband's aftershave to help soother barber's rash; diffuse in your teen's room when they are battling with exam stress or make a blend to help treat your tot's bronchitis.

Whilst aromatherapy is considered an alternative remedy, there has actually been a lot more research into the use of essential oils and the effects that they have then there has when it comes to modern medicines and drugs.

The ancient Egyptians got the ball rolling initially when it came to essential oils. They were the first culture to be able to effectively distill essential oils. They used these oils in religious ceremonies, as perfumes, in cosmetics and medicinally as well. The strongest cases for the efficacy of essential oils can be seen in the mummies that the ancients embalmed. Even thousands of years later, these bodies are in a reasonably good state of preservation thanks to the essential oils used during the embalming process. Even now, thousands of years later, the mummies still remain slightly fragrant thanks to the use of essential oils like Myrrh and Cedar Wood.

The oils were, in fact, so highly prized that the ancients used them frequently as offering to the gods. The priests in the temples were tasked with learning more about the healing properties of the oils and the secrets recipes that they learned were recorded.

One generation learned from the previous one and so it is not unreasonable to class aromatherapy as one of the earliest branches of medical research.

The ancient Romans also made extensive use of essential oils - Nero was well-known for his love of Rose oil - the oil that allowed him to continue with his highly social lifestyle.

And so it continued, with essential oils being adopted by most cultures around the globe. As the years passed, more and more research conducted into the use of these oils.

Modern aromatherapy was "rediscovered" by a Frenchman named Gattefosse. He was working in his family's perfumery lab one day when he burnt his hand quite severely. The only liquid nearby was a vat of Lavender oil and so he immediately put his hand into it.

When he realized that the burn was healing a lot faster than normal and that there was no blistering, he began to become obsessed with the healing benefits of essential oils and started more research into them.

A French woman, Marguerite Maury, developed the principles of conventional aromatherapy that we follow today - she researched effective methods of dilution and application through massage.

In the last couple of decades, there has been a resurgence in interest in natural remedies as we begin to realize that there are very real, negative long term side effects associated with synthetically-manufactured medications and products.

More and more evidence is surfacing that essential oils can be just as effective as more conventional treatments but without the negative side effects.

Why should you use aromatherapy? Well, the fact is that you probably already are to a small extent.

Essential oils are derived from various different parts of the plant - the petals, roots, bark, peel, fruit or resin. You may in contact with the same essences during the course of your day - take the lemon that you use for your detox drink. It is strongly scented and just through smelling the peel, you are benefiting from the essence of the plant itself.

You are basically giving yourself an aromatherapy treatment quickly and easily so why not go the whole hog and learn a bit more about using essential oils to your benefit?

Now, obviously the essential oil of a plant is a lot more concentrated than the essence that you get out of just one piece, but the idea is still the same.

# Chapter 2: How Aromatherapy and Works and its Use of Essential Oils

## The Chemistry of Aromatherapy and Essential Oils

Essential oils can be broken down into a range of different compounds such as ketones, esters, aldehydes, etc. The exact mixture of compounds is unique to the species of plant and have been produced by the plant to overcome potential evolutionary challenges.

Plants need protection against disease and help to thrive as much as we do and that is where the compounds that they produce come in.

The actual chemistry behind essential oils does become quite complex. It is not just one or two compounds that go into each oil but hundreds in most cases.

What makes essential oils so important as a curative treatment is that they are so easily able to cross the skin barrier and get to work in the blood stream. They are so effective at this that topical application or inhalation of the oils is, contrary to what you might think, a much more effective means of delivery than taking the oils internally would end up being.

## The Scientific Stuff

In general, essential oils consist of chemical compounds which have hydrogen, carbon and oxygen as their building blocks. These can be subdivided into two groups: the hydrocarbons which are made up almost exclusively of terpenes (monoterpenes, sesquiterpenes and diterpenes); and the oxygenated compounds, mainly esters, aldehydes, ketones, alcohols, phenols and oxides; acids, lactones, sulphur and nitrogen compounds are sometimes also present.

## Terpenes

Common terpene hydrocarbons include limonene (antiviral, found in 90 per cent of citrus oils) and pinene (antiseptic, found in high proportions in pine and turpentine oils); also camphene, cadinene, caryophyllene, cedrene, dipentene, phellandrene, terpinene, sabinene, and myrcene among others.

Some sesquiterpenes, such as chamazulene and farnesol (both found in Chamomile oil), have been the object of great interest recently due to their outstanding anti-inflammatory and bactericidal properties.

## Esters

Probably the most widespread group found in essential oils, which includes linalyl acetate (found in Bergamot, Clary Sage and Lavender), and geranyl acetate (found in Sweet Marjoram). They are characteristically fungicidal and sedative, often having a fruity aroma. Other esters include bornyl acetate, eugenyl acetate and lavendulyl acetate.

## Aldehydes

Citral, citronellal and neral are important aldehydes found notably in lemon-scented oils such as Melissa, Lemongrass,Lemon Verbena, Citronella etc. Aldehydes in general have a sedative effect; citral has been found to have specifically antiseptic properties. Other aldehydes include benzaldehyde, cinnamic aldehyde, cuminic aldehyde and perillaldehyde.

## Ketones

Some of the most common toxic constituents are ketones, such as thujone found in Mugwort, Tansy, Sage and Wormwood; and pulegone found in Penny Royal and Buchu – but this does not mean that all ketones are dangerous. Non-toxic ketones include jasmone found in Jasmine, and fenchone in Fennel oil. Generally considered to ease congestion and aid the flow of mucus, ketones are often found in plants which are used for upper respiratory complaints, such as hyssop and sage. Other ketones include camphor, carvone, menthone, methyl nonyl ketone and pinocamphone.

## Alcohols

One of the most useful groups of compounds, tending to have good antiseptic and antiviral properties with an uplifting quality; they are also generally non-toxic. Some of the most common terpene alcohols include linalol (found in Rosewood, Linaloe and Lavender), citronellol (found in Rose, Lemon, Eucalyptus and Geranium) and geraniol (found in Palmarosa); also borneol, menthol, nerol, terpineol, farnesol, vetiverol, benzyl alcohol and cedrol among others.

## Phenols

These tend to have a bactericidal and strongly stimulating effect, but can be skin irritants. Common phenols include eugenol (found in Clove and West Indian Bay), thymol (found in Thyme), carvacrol (found in Oregano and Savory); also methyl eugenol, methyl chavicol, anethole, safrole, myristicin and apiol among others.

# Oxides

By far the most important oxide is cineol (or eucalyptol) which stands virtually in a class of its own. It has an expectorant effect, well known as the principal constituent of Eucalyptus oil. It is also found in a wide range of other oils, especially those of a camphoraceous nature such as Rosemary, Bay Laurel, Tea Tree and Cajeput. Other oxides include linalol oxide found in hyssop (decumbent variety), ascaridol, bisabolol oxide and bisabolone oxide.

# The Harvesting of Essential Oils

As mentioned above, the oils are harvested from different sections of the plant. The tougher the plant material, the more robust the method of extraction should be. For example, Lavender stalks are quite tough and so need to be subjected to strong pressure in order to get the maximum amount of essential oils out.

Jasmine oil, on the other hand, is extracted from the flower petals and requires a more gentle approach - usually solvent extraction.

Some oils are a lot more difficult to harvest than others and produce a much smaller yield, making them a lot more expensive. Jasmine, for example, must be hand-picked, preferably when the flowers are no older than a day, for the best results. As you may only use the flowers, one plant will only produce a limited amount of oil.

The same can be said of roses where, again, only the rose petals are used to make the essential oil. One ton of rose petals is required to create just one pound of essential oil and so it is hardly surprising that Rose Otto oil is the most expensive or that the Rose oils found in stores are most likely to be a blend of Rose with less expensive oils.

On the other hand, some plants are very versatile when it comes to essential oils - take the orange, for example. Neroli oil is extracted from the flowers, Petitgrain oil from the leaves and Sweet Orange oil from the peel of the fruit.

## Essential Oil Vintages

As strange as it might sound, one "vintage" of essential oils may differ significantly from the next, depending upon growing conditions, climate, harvesting methods, etc. Just like you will have some years with exceptional vintages at a winery, you will have some years that the essential oil harvested will be exceptional. Unfortunately, there will also be years when the vintage is not that good.

That is where choosing a reputable company when choosing what essential oils to buy becomes essential. In the same way that you would place more trust in an experienced wine producer, you should place more trust in an experienced essential oil producer as well.

## How Essential Oils Are Extracted

The words "essential oil" tend to be bandied about a lot and are rather loosely applied to all aromatic products or extracts derived from natural sources, including concretes, resinoids and absolutes which contain a mixture of volatile and non-volatile components, such as wax or resin. This is not strictly accurate, since they are only partially composed of essential oils and are obtained by different methods of production, which include the use of solvents or more recently, carbon dioxide extraction. However, it is always the essential oil content in a given product that accounts for its aromatic quality.

Some plant materials, especially flowers, are subject to deterioration and should be processed as soon as possible after harvesting; others, including seeds and roots, are either stored or transported for extraction, often to Europe or America. The method of extraction which is employed depends on the quality of the material which is being used, and the type of aromatic product that is required.

## Essential Oils

An essential oil is extracted from the plant material by two main methods: by simple expression or pressure, as is the case with most of the citrus oils including Lemon and Bergamot, or by steam, water or dry distillation. The majority of oils such as Lavender, Myrrh, Sandalwood and Cinnamon are produced by steam distillation. This process only isolates the volatile and water-insoluble parts of a plant – many other (often valuable) constituents, such as tannins, mucilage and bitters are consequently excluded from the essential oil.

Sometimes the resulting oil is re-distilled or rectified to get rid of any remaining non-volatile matter; some essential oils are re-distilled at different temperatures to obtain certain constituents and exclude others – as with camphor which is split into three fractions, white, yellow and brown.

Essential oils are usually liquid, but can also be solid (orris) or semi-solid according to temperature (As is often the case with pure Rose oil). They dissolve in pure alcohol, fats and oils but not in water and, unlike the so-called 'fixed' plant oils (such as olive oil), they evaporate when exposed to air leaving no oily residue behind.

# Concretes

Concretes are prepared almost exclusively from raw materials of vegetable origin, such as the bark, flower, leaf, herb or root. The aromatic plant material is subjected to extraction by hydrocarbon-type solvents, rather than distillation or expression. This is necessary when the essential oil is adversely affected by hot water and steam, as is the case with Jasmine; it also produces a more true-to-nature fragrance.

Some plants, such as Lavender and Clary sage, are either steam distilled to produce an essential oil or used to produce a concrete by solvent extraction. The remaining residue is usually solid and of a waxy non-crystalline consistency.

Most concretes contain about 50%wax and 50% volatile oil, such as in the case of Jasmine; in rare cases, as with Ylang Ylang, the concrete is liquid and contains about 80% essential oil, 20% wax. The advantage of concretes is that they are more stable and concentrated than pure essential oils.

# Resinoids

Resinoids are prepared from natural resinous material by extraction with a hydrocarbon solvent, such as petroleum ether or hexane. In contradistinction to concretes, the resinoids are prepared from dead organic material, whereas concretes are derived from previously live tissue.

Typical resinous materials are balsams (Peru Balsam or Benzoin), resins (Mastic and Amber), oleoresins (Copaiba Balsam and Turpentine) and oleo gum resins (Frankincense and Myrrh). Resinoids can be viscous liquids, semi-solid or solid, but are usually homogeneous masses of non-crystalline character.

Occasionally the alcohol-soluble fraction of a resinoid is called an absolute.

Some resinous materials like Frankincense and Myrrh are used either to make an essential oil by steam distillation or a resin absolute by alcohol extraction directly from the crude oleo gum resin.

Benzoin, on the other hand, is insufficiently volatile to produce an essential oil by distillation: liquid Benzoin is often simply a Benzoin resinoid dissolved in a suitable solvent or plasticizing diluent.

Like concretes, resinoids are employed in perfumery as fixatives to prolong the effect of the fragrance.

## Absolutes

An absolute is obtained from the concrete by a second process of solvent extraction, using pure alcohol (ethanol) in which the unwanted wax is only slightly soluble. An absolute is usually subjected to repeated treatment with alcohol; even so, as is the case with orange flower absolute, a small proportion of the wax remains.

Absolutes can be further processed by molecular distillation which removes every last trace of non-volatile matter. The alcohol is recovered by evaporation which requires a gentle vacuum towards the end of the process. Some absolutes, however, will still retain traces of ethyl alcohol, at about 2%t or less, and are not recommended for therapeutic work because of these impurities.

Absolutes are usually highly concentrated viscous liquids, but they can in some cases be solid or semi-solid (Clary Sage absolute). In recent years, much research has been devoted to the extraction of essential oils and aromatic materials using liquid carbon dioxide;

oils produced in this manner are of excellent odor quality and are entirely free of unwanted solvent residues or non-volatile matter.

# Chapter 3: Your Aromatic First Aid Kit

## The Best Essential Oils to Have on Hand

There are hundreds of oils on the market - deciding which to keep at home can be a little confusing - after all, they are mostly good. It is tempting to want to buy as many different oils as you can but this is a mistake.

## Oils That Smell Good

For starters, there are going to be some oils that you like more than others and your preferences are not always going to match up with those of your family's. The truth is that if you do not like the smell of a particular oil, you just are not going to use it and it will end up going to waste - I still have a bottle of Patchouli oil somewhere at the back of one of my cupboards but I can't remember which one and I can't be bothered to look for it - I really dislike the smell.

Choose oils for your first aid kit based on what scents you like. Chances are that if you like Sandalwood, for example, you'll also like other oils in the wood family, like Cedar Wood.

## One Bottle Lasts For Ages

The second reason that I caution against buying too many bottles of oils is that you use so little at a time that one bottle will last you months. You will probably get tired of the scent before the bottle runs out.

Having a stash of 20 different oils may seem to make sense but if you consider that their shelf-life once opened is around 6 months to 2 years, it can also be a costly endeavour.

# Let's Make it Easy For You

To make things a little easier for you, I am going to list my top 10 oils for your first aid kit. The first three are oils that everyone should start off with. After that, pick and choose as it suits you.

## Lavender

This is one of the world's best-loved oils. I do find that the scent can be a bit overpowering in a blend but you can work around that. In my house, I always have a bottle of Lavender oil. (I have to, I am prone to burning myself - I have a love/ hate relationship with the oven, my glue gun and soldering iron - I love using them but they seem to hate me!)

Anyhow, Lavender oil is one of the gentlest oils that there is. It is safe to use on babies over the age of 10 weeks and can, in need, be applied neat to the skin. It is also one of the oils that is safe to use on your dogs and very useful in warding off ticks and fleas.

If you have small kids or are a keen gardener, you have to have Lavender oil. Mix up a bottle of the blend and keep it handy to deal with scratches, grazes, insect bites, minor cuts, allergic rashes, bruises and burns. Applied to chicken pox pustules, it can reduce infection and promote healing of the skin. It can help to soothe sunburn and to kill off lice.

It has analgesic properties and is also an anti-histamine so it can help to soothe allergic reactions and help to reduce pain as well. It is a strong antibacterial agent and can kill off fungi as well. It also helps skin to rejuvenate itself.

Diffuse when you have a bad cough or congested chest and it will help to soothe wheezing.

Used in a diffuser, it scents the room nicely and helps to calm frazzled nerves as well.

If you have a headache, a couple of drops massaged into the temples can help to shake it off.

If you have a migraine, massage a couple of drops into the temples and use in a cool compress behind the neck and over the eyes to help alleviate pain. If you are battling with nausea related to the migraine, rub some Lavender oil over the abdomen.

Tight muscles or sore joints can be eased by rubbing some of the oil into them directly or by adding a few drops to your bath water.

If you battle with insomnia, diffusing Lavender oil around about half an hour before bedtime while you are winding down can help your feel sleepy.

Alternatively, put a couple of drops onto your pillow.

Lavender is by far the most versatile oil and the one that has the most uses. It is relatively easy to find and not too expensive. It is classified as a "Middle" note and blends easily with just about every other oil. It is a definite must-have oil for any first aid kit.

## Eucalyptus Oil

Eucalyptus should definitely be a part of your kit if you are an athlete or avid sportsperson - it is really great for soothing stiff and sore muscles.

It is also essential if you have young kids or if you or anyone in your family is prone to getting respiratory tract infections.

Eucalyptus oil has quite a strong scent and has strong anti-bacterial and anti-viral properties. It is wonderful for unblocking a stuffy nose and relieving the symptoms and aches of cold and the flu. It is also great for getting rid of a sinus headache.

Rub a blend of Eucalyptus and Lavender oil into the feet at night to help the body fight infection and to help break a fever.

Used in a skin care blend, very diluted, it can also help to fight infections of the skin.

Diffuse it when sitting outside on the patio on the insects will leave you alone.

If you are battling with cellulite, a daily massage with a Eucalyptus blend will help detoxify and smooth skin and also boost circulation.

It is classified as a Top note when it comes to blending - meaning that the scent is one of the more volatile ones. It can be blended with Basil, Benzoin, Cedar Wood, Frankincense, Juniper, Lavender, Lemon, Marjoram, Melissa, Rosemary and Thyme.

# Chamomile

Chamomile oil is another one of those must-have oils. It does have a very sweet smell so you will either love it or be indifferent to it but it is also another of the gentle oils that can be used on babies over the age of 10 weeks.

It is the oil that has the strongest analgesic properties and it blends very well with Lavender to create a potent headache treatment. Just use as a cold compress applied to the back of the neck and rub a few drops of the blend into each temple.

If your baby is teething or if you have a tooth ache, Chamomile is very effective at relieving that throbbing pain. Apply a blend of Chamomile and Lavender to the outside of the mouth where the trouble is. A couple of drops massaged into the outside of the ear can help to soothe earache.

It will also help to reduce anxiety and stress - it is ideal to soothe a toddler who is battling with teething pains and can effectively put a stop to a temper tantrum.

It can relieve aching muscles and joints - it is a strong anti-inflammatory.

It is also a very effective anti-spasmodic as a topical treatment - use for menstrual cramping or stomach troubles.

It can help to soothe allergic skin reactions and eczema. It helps to soothe dry, troubled skin - mix with Lavender and Sandalwood for a wonderful treatment for skin that is suffering from exposure.

It is classified as a Middle note and will blend well with Benzoin, Bergamot, Clary Sage, Geranium, Jasmine, Lavender, Marjoram, Melissa, Patchouli, Rose and Ylang Ylang.

# Sandalwood

Sandalwood oil is one of the more expensive oils but a little really goes a long way. It is a superb fixative oil and blends well with many different oils. I have to admit that this is one of my favorite oils. I also find that I use it a lot. If the cost is too much for you, Cedar Wood oil has similar properties but is more affordable.

Sandalwood is particularly important if you have mature, dry skin. Mixed into a blend of Neroli, Palmrosa and Lavender, it is a potent anti-wrinkle treatment to use at night.

It is a great sinus cleanser and will help alleviate dry coughs and the symptoms of colds and the flu.

Where it really shines though is in its ability to help you to relax and relieve nervous tension, especially when these are a result of a fear of change.

As a fixative, there is no oil to match it. I once made a batch of aqueous cream, using Sandalwood as the fixative and no preservatives. The bottle rolled under a bookcase and I forgot about it. A couple of years later, we moved house and the bottle was found. The blend still smelled as good as it had on the day it was blended.

# Neroli

I love the smell of Neroli oil - it smells great and is a wonderful addition to any perfume blend.

Just a note of caution here though - when I was still working, a friend of mine and I decided that we needed a bit of a pick-me-up. We took a piece of cotton and added a few drops of Neroli. This we then put onto the radiator. The warmth from the radiator heated the oils and the scent permeated the room and very soon we were feeling great. We added a few more drops. After about an hour though, we were feeling a little to high-spirited and found just about everything funny. We had developed a mild buzz just from the Neroli oil! Granted, the room we were working in was pretty small and we had the windows closed to keep warm but this was one occasion when we had too much of a good thing.

If you are using the oil in a diffuser, make sure to use it for about a maximum of half an hour at a time. Alternatively, make sure that the room is properly ventilated. In all fairness, this never happened again and I use Neroli oil quite often in my perfume blends.

If you have a scar or stretch marks, this is a  great oil to have on hand - blended with Lavender and Geranium and Rose Hip oil, this is a wonderful treatment oil to encourage the reduction of scar tissue and to help regenerate skin.

Combined with Sandalwood it makes a perfect treatment for dry or dehydrated skin.

If you are battling with poor circulation, this is a good oil to use. It also has anti-spasmodic properties so can help relieve cramping.

If you have chronic diarrhoea or flatulence, rubbing a Neroli blend into the abdomen can provide much needed relief. It is particularly helpful in treating Irritable Bowel Syndrome.

It is a very uplifting oil and is effective in treating depression and nervous tension. Use a blend of Neroli when you are feeling especially anxious and it will calm you down very quickly.

Perhaps I am just biased because I love the scent of Neroli oil but it is one of the best oils for perfume. It is a citrus oil but does not smell overtly of citrus - to me it is more floral and sweet. It provides a great top note for a perfume blend. It blends well with most other oils but is especially good with Benzoin, Frankincense, Geranium, Lavender and Rose.

## Geranium

This is another of the oils that I always keep on hand. It is an inexpensive oil that is really great for the skin and so I often use it in blends. It is often used in Rose blends as it has similar properties to Rose oil and is said to smell like Rose oil. (Personally, to me it smells very different from Rose - it has a very herbaceous aroma.)

This does tend to overpower blends so I use 2 drops of any other oils in the blend for every 1 drop of Geranium oil.

The oil is a powerful skin healer and regenerator. For a particularly effective eczema treatment, get yourself an organic aqueous cream, some Geranium oil, some Palmrosa oil and Sandalwood oil. Used twice daily, this will clear up eczema and other allergic skin reactions.

There are no oils to beat Geranium when it comes to skin treatments - it helps to balance troubled skin and hydrate dry skin. Use on sunburned skin to reduce blistering and to soothe the burn. Apply to insect bites and allergic rashes for instant relief.

It is a good anti-inflammatory and so will reduce the appearance of red, raised pimples, prevent the infection of these, promote healing and reduce the chances of scarring.

I always mix up a bit of Lavender and Geranium oil whenever I am planning to do some crafting - it can be applied to cuts (my rotary cutter also hates me) and burns and will help them heal faster.

If you battle with water retention or cellulite, mix a few drops of oil into some olive oil and enough coarse salt to make a paste. Apply to the areas worst affected and then rinse off in a warm shower or soak off in a warm bath. Skin will feel smoother and softer and circulation will be boosted.

Geranium oil is said to have a balancing effect on the hormonal system and so can be useful if you suffer with premenstrual syndrome or if you are menopausal.

This is an uplifting oil that is useful in the treatment of depression and nervous tension.

It should not be used by pregnant women in their first trimester and should not be used by those diagnosed with breast or ovarian cancer.

This is classified as a Middle note and blends well with Basil, Bergamot, Grapefruit, Jasmine, Lavender, Neroli, Orange, Patchouli, Petitgrain, Rose, Rosemary, Sandalwood, Ylang Ylang.

# Ylang Ylang

If you want an oil that is truly exotic, this is it. You are either going to love it or hate it, there is no middle ground here. I love it but use it in limited quantities as it has quite a heady scent. If I feel a headache coming on, I avoid it as the strong scent can make a headache worse.

It is useful in balancing the sebum levels in the skin - making it suitable for use by people with all types of skin. Used in the rinse water after shampooing your hair, it helps increase shine and healthy hair.

It can be helpful at reducing high blood pressure and at regulating the heart.

It helps to reduce nervous tension and is renowned as an aphrodisiac. It can help to treat insomnia but I find that you need to be careful to use it in a blend here as the scent alone can end up being too strong. (I once sprinkled a few drops on my pillow to help me to sleep only to find that I needed to swap out my pillow because of the scent.)

What I find more effective is to mix 1 drop of Ylang Ylang, 1 drop Vetiver and 2 drops of Sandalwood and put them in the diffuser half an hour or so before bedtime. This is a very relaxing blend.

What I really love Ylang Ylang for is as a perfume oil - it rounds off sharp notes and can really take your perfume blend up to the next level. It also acts as a fixative in perfumes.

This is classified as a Base note and blends well with Grapefruit, Bergamot, Orange, Jasmine, Geranium, Sandalwood and Vetiver.

# Sweet Marjoram

This is not an oil that is commonly recommended in popular magazines, etc. and I think that this is such a pity. Whilst this is not an oil that I would use in perfumery because it has a strong scent, I do find that its other qualities more than make up for this.

I find that it is particularly useful for relieving tired and sore muscles and joints, especially if blended with a little Lavender oil. It warms the muscles and is very soothing overall.

If you battle with circulatory problems or high blood pressure, this is one oil that should be on your shopping list - it can help reduce bruising, regulate blood pressure and also prevent chilblains.

It has strong anti-bacterial and anti-viral properties making it useful in the treatment of colds and the flu. Mixed with Chamomile and Lavender oils, it makes a soothing rub for a tight chest and wracking cough.

It has anti-spasmodic properties and can be used in a warm compress to help alleviate menstrual cramps and pain. It helps to regulate the menstrual cycle, particularly when blended with Clary Sage.

For me personally, it is its calming effect that is most helpful. If I find that I am feeling panicky or over-anxious, Sweet Marjoram blended with either Lime or Chamomile always helps me put things back into perspective.

Mixed with Lavender and Chamomile, this makes a really effective treatment for headaches and migraines - massage into the temple or use as a cool compress over the forehead and at the back of the neck .

# Peppermint

I'm pretty sure that you have heard about the digestion soothing effects of Peppermint tea. The essential oil is equally as useful but also has a few uses that you may not have known about.

Peppermint's regulating effects on the digestive system make it a truly useful herb and one that does deserve a place in the top ten. It can help to ease dyspepsia, indigestion, colic and flatulence.

It also has strong anti-spasmodic properties making it a valuable addition to a post-workout blend. In addition, is aids circulation, warms muscles and soothes aches in muscles and joints.

I do avoid using the oil on my face though and do only use it at a maximum of 1% dilution as it may cause irritation to the skin.

I find that the oil is especially useful in the treatment of head colds - there is nothing better to clear up a nasty sinus infection than a blend of Peppermint, Eucalyptus and Lavender oils.

I use this oil a lot when I need to focus - it is a very stimulating oil and clears out foggy thinking very fast. It should not be used near to bedtime as it can keep you awake.

It can also interfere with the efficacy of homeopathic treatments and should never be used by pregnant women.

## Rosemary

Rosemary is another of those scents that you will either love or hate. It is quite a strong scent and can be overpowering in a blend so again, use 2 drops of your other oils with every 1 drop of Rosemary oil.

This is one oil that is very good for oily skin and is useful in the treatment of acne. It is too harsh for dry or sensitive skin though. It is a great oil to help stimulate hair growth - rub a blend of Rosemary and Lavender into the scalp just about half an hour before washing your hair to help promote hair growth and a healthy scalp. (Preferably not within 2-3 hours of bedtime).

It is a very effective stimulant for the circulatory system and warms muscles. It has analgesic properties so is particularly good for those suffering from muscle stiffness and soreness, especially when this is due to overwork. It can also be valuable in relieving arthritic and rheumatic pain.

Rosemary oil is a good tonic for the liver and gallbladder so rub over the abdomen after over-indulging.

Rosemary oil is very effective at treating disorders of the respiratory system such as sinusitis and bronchitis. Blend with eucalyptus to ease coughing and wheezing.

Rosemary is also very useful in the treatment of headaches, especially if these are brought on by stress and tension. Apply as a cool compress to the back of the neck.

In ancient times, Roman soldiers would tuck a sprig of Rosemary behind their ears to help them focus their attention. This tactic is just as effective when using Rosemary oil. When I really need to focus on writing or studying, I blend together Rosemary oil and Lime oil and massage it into my scalp. I find that this helps me to focus for longer periods of time and let's me work longer and harder, with less chance of fatigue setting in.

Rosemary is classified as a Middle note and blends well with Basil, Bergamot, Frankincense, Geranium, Grapefruit, Lavender, Lemongrass, Lime, Mandarin, Orange, Pine and Petitgrain.

These are the 10 oils that I find most useful. With the exception of the first three, which should be part of every essential oil first aid kit, I encourage you to pick and choose oils that you think will be most useful to you.

Start off with the three essential essential oils and see how that goes. If you enjoy practising aromatherapy, add a few of the other oils in the list. There is no rush to build up the ultimate collection of oils - add them as and when your budget allows you to.

Here is a quick break down of which oils to use for what (there may be some overlap - some oils fall into several categories:

**Analgesics:** Analgesics relieve pain. Good oils in this category include Peppermint, Black Pepper, Chamomile, Sweet Marjoram, Rosemary and Juniper. Clove can also be used if well-diluted and in moderation.

**Anti-Inflammatory:** Anti-inflammatory oils reduce swelling. Good oils in this category include Eucalyptus, Peppermint, Tea Tree, Chamomile, Lavender, Frankincense, Myrrh.

**Anti-Septics:** These oils clean wounds and help to prevent infection. Good oils in this category include Bergamot, Tea Tree, Lemon, Lavender, Rosemary, Thyme, Frankincense, Sandalwood, Benzoin, Ginger.

**Immune Stimulants:** These oils help to build up immunity and to speed recovery. Good oils in this category include Tea Tree, Geranium, Lavender, Rosemary, Frankincense, Clove.

# Chapter 4: Bathing for Better Health

## The Benefits of Combining Aromatherapy and Hydrotherapy

The ancient Romans understood the importance of hydrotherapy. A trip to the baths was about more than just personal hygiene and could last a few hours - it was a place to relax and unwind, to discuss business and even a place to improve physical fitness.

The idea was to induce sweating by moving through a series of rooms, each one hotter than the last. Most public baths would have the same set up. You would start in an Apodyterium, the ancient equivalent of a locker room. Next up would be a visit to the Frigidarium, the cold room which had a bath of cold water. After than you would moved to a Tepidarium, a room that was warmer. The final room in the series, the Caldarium was the hottest room and was always heating using a brazier. There were usually basins containing cool water to allow you to cool off in need.

You would generally round everything off by having a massage using essential oils. The oils would be scraped off and you would either proceed to the Laconium to rest, if there was one, or back to the Apodyterium to get dressed and be on your way.

These ancient baths formed the basis for what we would now call a modern spa and the treatment potential is just as important now as it was back then.

Whilst today we may not have the time to spend the whole morning in the bath, a quick session in the sauna can produce benefits as well.

For those who have no access to a sauna, a bath or shower will do just as well. Cranking up the hot water in the bath or shower and letting the steam clear your senses is as therapeutic as sitting in a sauna.

## Essential Oils in the Bath

Essential oils can help you elevate the treatment potential of your bath exponentially. And it is so easy - simply draw your bath and add in a few drops of the essential oils of your choice just before you climb in. It really couldn't be simpler.

The oils themselves will not diffuse in the water but the heat from the water will help the oils to evaporate - that is why you should only add them after the bath has been drawn.

It is important to add, at the very most, 6 drops of essential oils in a full bath because of the potential to irritate the skin. What I advise is to start with no more than two drops of one particular oil and to note the reaction to your skin. Add another oil in a different session and you will quickly find which oils irritate the skin and which do not.

The key to avoiding irritation is to be careful about the number of oils added - bath time is not the time to try complex blends and to limit your bath to no longer than 20 or 30 minutes at most.

Irritation does not necessarily mean that you will develop a rash - your skin may become red, tingly or intensely itchy. If this happens, get out of the bath, dry yourself off and apply an aqueous cream to the affected areas.

I usually find though that simply drying myself off is often enough to get rid of any irritation.

Of course, there are other ways to reduce irritation in the bath.

# Bath to Beat Colds and the Flu

2 Drops Eucalyptus oil

2 Drops Juniper oil

2 Drops Sweet Orange oil

2 Cups Epsom Salts (Optional)

½ Cup Baking Soda (Optional)

The Epsom Salts and Baking Soda should be left out if you have high blood pressure or are pregnant.

Run a hot bath, adding the Epsom Salts and Baking Soda while drawing the bath so that they dissolve. Just before climbing into the bath, add your oils. Relax for at least 20 minutes. Dry yourself off and wrap up warmly when you are finished in the bath. This bath will detox your system and cause you to sweat the virus out.

# Restore the Skin's pH Balance

2 Drops Geranium oil

2 Drops Sandalwood oil

1 cup Apple Cider Vinegar

Draw a tepid bath. Mix the oils with the Apple Cider vinegar and add to the bath just before you climb in. Soak for at least 20 minutes.

# Add the Oils to Some Full-Fat Milk

Oils will not diffuse in water but the fat in the milk helps them to do just that. Use about a cup of milk and, again, no more than 6 drops of essential oil. Mix the two together and then add to the bath just before getting in. Swirl the water to mix in the milk.

This has the added benefit of being good for your skin as well. It is said that Cleopatra used to bath in asses' milk to keep her skin young and supple and modern research shows that there may be some truth in that - the lactic acid in the milk can help to slough off dead skin cells and so help to soften skin.

## Beauty Bath Fit for a Queen (or King)

2 Drops Sandalwood oil

2 Drops Ylang Ylang oil

2 Drops Neroli oil

1 Cup Full-fat milk

Draw a tepid bath - in this case the bath water should not be too hot. Mix the essential oils into your milk. Just before you get into the bath, add the milk mixture and swirl the water so that it is properly incorporated. Relax for about 20 minutes.

## Itchy Skin Relief

2 Drops Lavender oil

2 Drops Geranium oil

2 Drops Palmrosa oil

1 Cup oatmeal

1 Cup milk

a Few sprigs Lavender flowers (if you have them in the garden)

A muslin bag

Place the oatmeal in the muslin bag and hang it under the hot tap as you are drawing your bath. The bath water should be tepid rather than hot. Once the bath has been drawn, toss the oatmeal bag into it.

Mix the oils and the milk and then add to the bath just before climbing into it.

Use the muslin bag with the oatmeal in it as a sponge, concentrating on the itchy areas.

## Add the Oils to Your Body First

Another option is to blend your chosen oils into a carrier oil and to massage them into your skin before you get into the bath. I find that this is particularly effective when it comes to relieving muscular aches and pains and is a great way to reduce skin irritation.

For full benefits, massage the blend into the areas as necessary and allow to settle for at least 15-20 minutes before climbing into a bath that is as warm as you can manage. The heat of the water helps to further increase the absorption of any excess oils and also helps to relieve soreness as well.

## After Sport's Rub

3 Drops Rosemary oil

2 Drops Lemon Grass oil

50ml Jojoba oil

Mix oils into oil, ensuring that they are well incorporated. Massage into sore muscles and leave in place for at least 20 minutes. Draw a hot bath and soak for at least 20 minutes.

# Using a Foot Bath

Perhaps you do not have a bath in your home, or perhaps you simply do not want to go to all the trouble of drawing one. A foot bath can be an effective alternative, especially when it comes to relieving the symptoms of colds and the flu.

Simply select a basin that is big enough to accommodate both feet and half-fill with warm water.

Add in the oils of your choice and soak your feet for at least 15-20 minutes.

## Golf Ball Foot Relief

I use this remedy of I have had to stand for long periods of time and I find that it is particularly effective for sore feet.

You will need:

A basin big enough to fit your feet in

2 Golf balls

1 Drop Lavender oil

1 Drop Eucalyptus oil

1 Drop Peppermint oil

2 Agapanthus leaves (optional)

Half-fill the basin with water as hot as you can manage. If using the agapanthus leaves, place them at the bottom of the basin. Place the golf balls into the basin as well and and then add in the oils. Soak your feet in the water, every now and again rolling your soles over the golf balls - this helps to relieve muscular tension in the feet.

Soak for about 20 minutes. If using the agapanthus leaves, wrap them around your feet and then wrap them with a towel, elevate your feet and leave the leaves in place for about 20 minutes. The use of warmed agapanthus leaves to alleviate foot aches is an old Zulu remedy - I realize that it sounds weird but it really does work.

Unwrap the leaves and dry off your feet. Apply a rich aqueous cream and socks and leave on for at least 20 minutes or, if possible, overnight.

# Using Hot/ Cold Water Combos

One of the most effective treatments when it comes to boosting circulation is to use hot and cold water alternatively. There are a couple of ways that you can do this at home - either in the shower or in the bath.

## In the Shower

After your normal shower, turn the tap to as cold as you can manage for about 2 minutes and then switch back to warm water again for about two minutes. Repeat a couple of times. This is a great way to boost circulation, rev up the metabolism, wake you up and firm up the skin in the areas concerned. Always end on a warm note.

# Power Shower

2 Drops Peppermint oil

2 Drops Rosemary oil

1 Clean wash cloth

Dampen the wash cloth and add the oils to it. Turn on the shower and place the wash cloth at your feet. The heat of the shower will release the scent of the oils and you will feel invigorated. Finish off with blasts of cold and warm water to really wake you up.

# Breast Firming Shower

2 Drops Neroli oil

2 Drops Rose oil blend

2 Drops Jasmine oil blend

60ml Rose Hip oil

This time we are not going to use the oils until after your shower. Alternate hot and cold a of water, concentrating on the breast area. Climb out of the shower and dry the skin on the breasts and decolletage. Apply the Rose Hip oil and essential oil blend and leave to soak in while you dry the rest of your body. Mop up any excess oil with a clean wash cloth or tissue.

# Sitz Bath

Whilst the ancient Romans had the luxury of being able to plunge into a cool bath of water after being in very hot room, most of us cannot boast the same luxury. A sitz bath is a good alternative and can be very effective but it is not suitable if you have high blood pressure or suffer from epilepsy.

You will need two basins large enough to sit in. Half fill one basin with very warm water and the other basin with very cold water. The idea is to sit in one basin and then put your feet in the other basin and stay this way for about 5 minutes before switching. Do this at least twice. Be warned, this is not for the faint-hearted - that cold basin will be a shock to the system, but that is the whole point, after all.

It is a good way to boost immunity, boost circulation and improve lymph drainage so it is worth persevering.

## Anti-Thrush/ Cystitis Sitz Bath

2 Drops Bergamot oil

2 Drops Sandalwood oil

Place oils in warm bath just before climbing into it. Soak for five minutes before switching baths. Repeat at least twice.

# Chapter 5: Cleansing the Air with Essential Oils

## Your Guide to a Cleaner and Healthier Home Environment

Essential oils are very effective when diffused or vaporised. The compounds within the oils delicately scent the air and also kill off germs in the atmosphere at the same time, leaving your home smelling better and also helping to curb the spread of diseases. All essential oils have anti-bacterial properties so you can choose just about any oils that you like to scent your home.

Where you do need to take care is when you are pregnant, epileptic, have young children or pets (Birds are especially sensitive to the effects of oils). Not all oils are safe in these instances. Rosemary, for example, can stimulate uterine contractions and thus cause early delivery. It can also bring on epileptic seizures in sufferers. It is also not one of the oils that is safe for use on children under the age of 5 years old and is not safe for use on your pets.

If any of the above conditions apply in your home, do take a little time to research a bit more about the safety of the oils that you are planning to use. Oils like Lavender and Chamomile are safe for young children, pregnant women, epileptics, dogs and cats.

Fortunately a little research online will be all you need to tell you whether or not the oils are safe to use all round.

# Better Than Chemicals

There are a lot of advantages to using diffused oils in place of synthetic air fresheners. At least we know that the essential oils are better for us to use. The synthetic air fresheners tend to smell fake and are packed with unhealthy chemicals.

The anti-bacterial qualities of the oil mean that they can also pack quite a punch when it comes to cleaning time. The best oils to vaporize in order to kill germs are: Bergamot, Citronella, Lavender, Lemon, Peppermint, Pine, Rosemary and Tea Tree.

Some oils also have insect-repellent qualities that are quite useful. Bergamot, Citronella, Eucalyptus and Peppermint are examples of these. In fact, if ants are a problem in your home, Peppermint added to the water used to wash your floors with will go a long way to repelling them. Citronella diffused into the air will chase away mosquitoes and flies.

# Cost Effective

The scent of the essential oils lingers longer and you use only a few drops at a time, making essential oils an attractive option financially.

# Easy to Use

All you need to do is to either pop a few drops of oil into a diffuser or aromatherapy burner, into a bowl of warm water near the radiator or mix it into a spray bottle and spritz the room - it could not be easier.

# Chapter 6: Steaming Your Way to Success With Essential Oils

## Harnessing Steam Treatments

When it comes to the use of essential oils, steam treatments and vaporization are ideal ways to get the full benefit of the oils without actually coming into direct contact with them at all. This is of especial benefit when you want to help ease breathing, calm the mind and is an effective beauty treatment as well.

## Vaporization

This is a great way to scent the rooms of your home, without worrying about the smoky atmosphere created by incense. Oils are vaporized by heating them up and causing them to diffuse into the air in your home.

An aromatherapy burner or diffuser are ideal methods of delivery, especially if you plan to make use of the therapy often. As an alternative, and if you still use incandescent light bulbs. you can look for a ceramic ring that fits on top of the bulb. You then add a few drops of oil to the ring and it is warmed by the bulb. If you have a radiator or use a heater or fire in winter, you can just fill a bowl with water and drop some oils into that. Keep the bowl in close proximity to the heat source and they will evaporate. Adding a bowl of water can also help to replace the humidity in a room when a heater is used.

Oils have long been used in rituals to create a specific ambience - Frankincense is traditionally used for promoting relaxation and reflectiveness of mind.

Oils can also be vaporized in order to clear off unpleasant odors like cigarette smoke and oils such as Lemongrass and Citronella have a firm value when it comes to being insect repellents.

In ancient medicinal texts, the burning of Rosemary and Juniper leaves was recommended to cleanse the air and to prevent the spread of infection. Rosemary is too stimulating to use at night so you can choose Eucalyptus oil or Myrtle oil in its place in the sickroom at night. Both are very effective at clearing congestion and easing breathing.

It is important to keep any aromatherapy burners out of the reach of children and pets - dogs may lap up the water or knock over the burner causing problems. Kids may do the same.

## Steam Inhalation

When you are ill and battling congestion, there is nothing better to clear out the mucous and the germs than a steam treatment. This is easily accomplished - all you need is to fill a bowl with hot water, add around about 5 drops of your chosen oil and to bend over the bowl and drape a towel over both your head and the bowl.

This creates a mini-steam chamber. Inhale deeply to allow the sinuses to unblock and to ensure that the vapor is drawn deep into the body so that germs and viruses are killed.

Stay in your "steam room" for at least 5-10 minutes so that the sinuses have a good chance to clear. You can alternatively use a hot bath though the effect is not as concentrated. This treatment is not recommended if you have high blood pressure or are an epileptic.

## Anti-Flu Steam Treatment

2 Drops Eucalyptus oil

2 Drops Peppermint oil

1 Drop Lavender oil

Add the oils to the steaming water and drape the towel around the head and breathe in deeply until the sinuses clear.

## Cold and Cough Steam Treatment

2 Drops Juniper Berry oil

1Drop Rosemary oil

2 Drops Lime oil

Add the oils to the steaming water and drape the towel around the head and breathe in deeply until the sinuses clear.

# Steam Treatment for a Bad Cough That Just Won't Quit

2 Drops Frankincense oil

2 drops Myrrh oil

2 Drops Bergamot oil

Add the oils to the steaming water and drape the towel around the head and breathe in deeply until the sinuses clear.

# Steam Treatment for Hay Fever and Asthma

2 Drops Eucalyptus oil

2 Drops Lavender oil

Add the oils to the steaming water and drape the towel around the head and breathe in deeply until the sinuses clear. Steam treatments are great for Hayfever as they clear the passageways and can help to humidify the mucous membrane of the nose and lungs.

# Steam Treatments for Beauty

Steam treatments can be helpful when it comes to unblocking your pores and livening up a dull complexion. If you have dry or sensitive skin or thread veins, you should avoid steam treatments for beauty purposes.

Basically, all you need is to fill a bowl with hot water, add around about 5 drops of your chosen oil and to bend over the bowl and drape a towel over both your head and the bowl. Steam the skin in this manner for about 5 minutes or so, once or twice a week at most. When finished, wipe the face with a wash cloth that has been soaked in warm, clean water to remove debris that has come to the surface of the skin and follow up by splashing the skin with cool water to help close the pores again. Pat skin dry and apply either Witch Hazel or Rose Water before moisturizing.

You can also find special facial saunas that make this process easier but these are not essential.

# Steam Treatment for Oily Skin

2 Drops Juniper oil

2 Drops Lavender oil

Add the oils to the steaming water and drape the towel around the head. Stay in position for about 5 minutes. When finished, wipe the face with a wash cloth that has been soaked in warm, clean water to remove debris that has come to the surface of the skin and follow up by splashing the skin with cool water to help close the pores again. Pat skin dry and apply either Witch Hazel or Rose Water before moisturizing.

# Steam Treatment for Cleansing Pores

2 Drops Lemon oil

2 Drops Tea Tree oil

Add the oils to the steaming water and drape the towel around the head. Stay in position for about 5 minutes. When finished, wipe the face with a wash cloth that has been soaked in warm, clean water to remove debris that has come to the surface of the skin and follow up by splashing the skin with cool water to help close the pores again. Pat skin dry and apply either Witch Hazel or Rose Water before moisturizing.

# Steam Treatment for Balancing Skin

2 Drops Jasmine/ Rose oil

2 Drops Lavender oil

1 Drop Geranium oil

Add the oils to the steaming water and drape the towel around the head. Stay in position for about 5 minutes. When finished, wipe the face with a wash cloth that has been soaked in warm, clean water to remove debris that has come to the surface of the skin and follow up by splashing the skin with cool water to help close the pores again. Pat skin dry and apply either Witch Hazel or Rose Water before moisturizing.

# Chapter 7: Make Your Own Signature Scent with Essential Oils

## Creating a One-of-a-Kind Perfume

Creating a perfume is about more than just mixing oils that you like and hoping for the best. When one oil is blended with another, a chemical reaction takes place and the entire nature of the blend is changed. Get it right and you have a wonderful aroma, get it wrong and the results can be disastrous - at best, a bland scent that has no personality and, at worst, a scent that is really awful.

The key to blending the different essential oils is to choose oils that compliment each other and that have compounds that work together with one another. I will go more into creating a healing synergy in the next chapter so for now it is enough to simply determine which oils work well together and which ones do not.

Of course, it is most important to find oils that you like to start out with. I like Ylang Ylang in a perfume, for example, but it is too sweet for my mother and it irritates her if I wear it around her. Everyone is different and so it pays to establish which oils you like.

If possible, find a store that provides testers of the oils so that you can sniff them before committing to buying one. Also be prepared to devote some time to this pursuit. What I advise is reading through this chapter and identifying two to three blends, each consisting of three oils, that you think you may like. (Your blends should match in terms of Fragrance Families and each should have a Top note, a Middle note and a Base note).

Write down the oils that you want to try and take this with you to the store. Ideally speaking, there should be strips of papers to drop the oils onto, if not, tear up strips of paper to take with you.

Starting with your first three oils, do your first smell test. Sniff the oil straight out of the bottle - if you do not like the smell out of the bottle, move on to the next oil.

If you do like the smell out of the bottle, place a drop of the oil on your paper strip - each oil should be on a different strip. Leave it for about 15 minutes and then sniff the strip. The character of the scent should have mellowed slightly. What do you think of it now?

Now combine two of the strips and see how you like that blend. Now add in the third. By now you will have a good idea of what the end blend will smell like and you should be able to choose your own oils.

I advise doing tests on no more than two blends a day as this can overpower the olfactory senses and lead to less than perfect results. Take your time, you are worth the little bit of extra effort.

I worked on getting my signature scent right for months. When I got the formula exactly right though, that effort was well worthwhile. Now all I need to do is to do is apply it and I instantly feel calmer and happier - it is like bottled happiness for me.

## Like With Like

In general, oils of the same botanical family blend well together. Also those which share common constituents usually mix well, such as the camphoraceous oils containing a good percentage of cineol, which includes all the members of the Myrtaceae group (Eucalyptus oil, Tea Tree oil, Cajeput oil, Myrtle oil, etc.) but also many herbs including Lavender, Rosemary and Spanish Sage.

Most floral fragrances blend well together, as do the woods, balsams, citrus oils and spices, etc. Rosewood and Linaloe, for example, combine well together, although they belong to different botanical families, since they both contain a high proportion of linalol and linalyl acetate.

Some oils such as Rose oil, Jasmine oil, Oakmoss oil and Lavender oil seem to enhance just about any blend, and are commonly found, to some extent, in commercial perfumes - though usually highly adulterated.

Some combinations, on the other hand, have an inhibiting power over one another. Essences with a predominance of aldehydes (such as Citronella oil containing citronellal), those with mainly ketones (such as Sage containing thujone) and those with high amounts of phenols (such as Clove oil containing eugenol), when combined with each other tend to 'pull' in different directions.

However, do not get to hung up on the exact chemical composition of the oils being used - start off by making up the blends I have shared with you until you start getting a feel for what makes a good blend. As you get more familiar with the character of each different oil, you will start to be able to instinctively know what goes well together.

Another thing to look at is the basic qualities of the oils in questions. An oil like Rosemary, for example, that is a very stimulating oil, will not pair well with an oil like Vertiver, a very relaxing oil. Look for oils with properties that compliment one another to get the right blend.

# Fragrance Families

When it comes to blending perfumes, it is important to understand the different fragrance families. Oils within the same fragrance family will blend together well. There are also some very well-known combinations between fragrance families that can be relied on when it comes to creating a blend with depth.

The spice and citrus oils, for example, are one such example of a good mix. The citrus and wood oils are another.

You can often create an interesting note by adding in a bit of an opposite family of scent but this is best left until you get the hang of blending.

Here are the basic fragrance families and some of the oils contained therein to get you started. Getting to know what fragrance family you like is also helpful when choosing oils in future. I prefer the Floral and Woody oils but am not fond of the Green tones, for example. My mother, on the other hand, likes the clean fresh Citrus scents and also the Green tones.

**Green:** Basil, Chamomile, Clary Sage, Eucalyptus, Galbanum, Pine, Rosemary, Spruce and Thyme

**Spicy:** Camphor, Fennel, Ginger, Juniper, Laurel, Sweet Marjoram, Myrrh, Tarragon and Tea Tree

**Floral:** Geranium, Jasmine, Lavender, Mimosa, Neroli, Rose, Rosewood, Violet and Ylang Ylang.

**Citrus:** Bergamot, Citronella, Grapefruit, Lemon, Lemongrass, Lime, Mandarin, Orange and Petitgrain.

**Woody/ Balsamic:** Ambrette, Angelica, Bay, Birch, Cedar Wood, Frankincense, Marigold, Patchouli, Sandalwood, Valerian and Yarrow.

# Perfumery is an Art

Whilst there is some science in terms of what compounds blend well together, creating the perfect blend is something of an art and should be approached as such. Just as you would in any other art form, you need to pay attention to composition here. Perfumery goes one step above the more traditional art forms though - a great blend not only smells wonderful but also evokes powerful positive emotions in those who smell it. It helps to improve mood and helps with relaxation. It can also be sensual and flirty, or fun, or exotic - depending on what the wearer prefers.

You are going to blend a few different oils together to create a scent that has depth but that is, at the same time, seamless. You will pick up notes of each scent but, if you get it right, the combination of scents will be unique and will add up to more than simply a sum of each separate oil.

Perfumers tend to use three or four dominant scents to make up the basic blend. They then add in small amounts of other scents in order to play with the final composition and to tweak it so that it is something really special.

Over time, you will start to get a feel for what oils blend well and what oils do not. Go with your instincts and don't be afraid to experiment a bit, you might be pleasantly surprised at the results. The absolute worst that can happen is that you hate the blend and need to throw it out and start all over again.

## The Top, Base, and the Middle

In order to get a balanced blend, it is important to have a top note, a base note and a middle note. All essential oils can be classified into one category or another, depending on how volatile they are.

**The Top Note:** These notes are the lightest and most volatile. These are the scent that you smell upon applying the blend and the scent that will wear off the fastest. Examples of top notes include Tea Tree oil, Eucalyptus oil, Mandarin oil, Lemon oil , Basil oil Bergamot oil, Neroli oil and Jasmine oil. Most of your citrus oils will fit in here.

**The Middle Note:** These are the "bulky" notes and will be at the heart of your scent. This scent is not immediately apparent and will also wear off quite quickly. Middle notes are not as volatile as top notes. Examples of middle notes include Geranium oil, Lavender oil, Sweet Marjoram oil, Rosewood oil and Rosemary oil. A lot of your herbal oils will fit in here.

**The Base Notes:** These are a rich, and lingering scents that are slow to emerge but long lasting. These notes are stable enough to help to anchor the more volatile oils and to prevent them from evaporating too fast. Examples of base notes include Patchouli oil, Rose oil, Jasmine oil, Benzoin oil, Frankincense oil, Myrrh oil, Sandalwood oil and Vetiver oil. Many of your spice oils and wood oils will fit into this category.

Ylang Ylang is one oil that can fulfil each of the the above-mentioned functions in a blend. It is considered a completely balanced oil.

When making your blend, start with the basic base note, the middle note and the top note. You will often find that you need less of the base note than the others as it has such a rich scent.

Add your oils in drop by drop - finding the right balance can be tricky and even just one drop out of place can make it necessary to re-balance the whole blend.

Once you are satisfied with the basic notes and how they are blended, then you can consider adding additional oils to create interest and depth.

# Keep a Record

Who knows, you might even hit on the next classic scent like Chanel No. 5. Imagine if you go through all that effort and then are unable to remember the oils that you used or the quantities of each oil.

Write down what oils you are using as you are adding them and make sure to also note changes in scent, etc. that appealed to you.

I don't care how bright you are, if you do not write it down, or, keep a video log, there is a better than average chance that at some stage you will want to recreate a blend and not be able to remember which oils went in to it.

Professional perfumers can recognise thousands of scents but it takes years and years to get that good. I have been experimenting with essential oils for over two decades now and, whilst I am pretty good at recognizing a scent on its own, and may even be able to distinguish scents where two oils have been blended together, anything more than that is beyond me.

The scents, especially when you make a great blend, will blend together to such an extent that they are chemically altered and a new scent is created. You may pick up a hint of one oil or the other, but rather don't take a chance, write everything down.

Besides, let's say that you do hit on the next big scent and it sells millions and millions of bottles making you an overnight success (dream big!), you will need your notes for when you write your autobiography.

My two biggest tips on getting your blending perfect?

Keep a written record and label your bottles so that you know what is in them.

# Chapter 8: Creating a Healing Synergy with Essential Oils

## How to Blend Aromatherapy Oils to Best Effect

Essential oils are blended mainly for two reasons - for their medicinal properties or to create a perfume.

When we are using pure essential oils, these are not two different categories but rather two ends of a scale. At one end of the scale we are dealing with the therapeutic action on a purely physical condition such as backache – at the other end, with an emotional or aesthetic response to a particular odor. But, of course, the individual who is suffering from lumbago also has a psychic or emotional disposition of which they may or may not be aware, which will naturally respond in a more subtle way to a particular blend of oils.

Let's say, for example, the smell of Eucalyptus brings up memories of a fun vacation to Australia for you. You will then no doubt enjoy using Eucalyptus oil. Someone else, on the other hand, may have had to use Eucalyptus oil when they were very ill and so their emotional associations to the oil may be quite different.

Now, thinking about it logically for a minute, and understanding the immense impact that our minds have on our ability to heal ourselves, how well do you think that Eucalyptus oil would work for someone who has such negative associations with it?

The basic compounds in the oil remain unchanged but using the oil may cause stress emotionally and so healing will be negatively affected.

# Manly Medicine

Another consideration is whether or not the fragrance will appeal to both sexes. There are not a lot of men that relish the idea of running around with a floral scent and so you may need to tailor the blend accordingly, skipping the Jasmine and choosing a more appropriate scent.

Once again, the key here is the emotional impact of the blend. Whilst a blend made up of floral oils will have the same components, no matter who is using it, it's efficacy on a particular person can be strongly influenced by what their perceptions of the appropriateness of the scent are.

# Creating Synergies

The proportions of each essential oil in a blend can also be vital to the effectiveness of the remedy as a whole (many aromatherapy books contain exact recipes for specific disorders).

Some oils blended together have a mutually enhancing effect upon one another, so that the whole is greater than the sum of the parts: for example, the anti-inflammatory action of chamomile is supported by being mixed with lavender.

When the blended oils are working harmoniously together, then the combination is called a 'synergy'. 'In order to create a good synergy, you must take into account not only the symptom to be treated but also the underlying cause of the disorder and the psychological or emotional factors involved.

This is very much the conclusion that Madame Maury reached when she prescribed individual prescriptions for each of her patients. She made sure that the blended essences were matched not only to their physical requirements, but also to their circumstances and temperament.

Someone who is suffering from intense anxiety, for example, should be paired with an oil that is grounding and relaxing like Vertiver oil. You would avoid using an oil like Rosemary, for example, as it is a very stimulating one.

# Chapter 9: Base Basics

## Creating a Firm Foundation for Your Treatments

Earlier in this book we have dealt with using essential oils in the bath or in a diffuser. The one constant is that essential oils should never be applied neat to the skin, with the exception of Lavender and Tea Tree oils. Because essential oil are so concentrated, applying them neat to the skin could result in a negative reaction and damage to your skin.

Fortunately, because the oils are so concentrated, you really do not need much to get the full benefit of the healing effects.

If you are going to be using the essential oils in beauty treatments or in healing remedies, you also need to know how to mix them with the right bases to get the best possible results.

Whilst you can mix essential oils into just about any oily base, there is definitely something to be said for choosing a base that is, in itself, a healing treatment. In this chapter I will speak about blending oils into an aqueous cream base and blending them into a number of different curative oils.

If you do not like the feel of oil on your skin, use a cream base - you can boost its curative properties by blending in some special oils at a 10% concentration - this gives you the benefit of the oils whilst still leaving you with a creamy, lighter texture.

# Aqueous Base

An aqueous cream is very simply a cream that has fewer ingredients - it is very moisturizing and is usually not colored or scented. These creams are ideal for people who battle with allergies and sensitive skin.

The bland base cream is ideal to add essential oils to so get yourself a fair amount of it, especially if you are going to start making your own body lotions.

Take some time and source an organic cream - it really is worth paying a bit extra here as the organic-based creams are a lot richer and more nourishing and tend to hold up better than the standard ones.

If you are serious about anti-aging or skin treatments, take the time to get an organic supplier. We have one that is about a half an hour's drive away so I buy a liter or two at a time. Our supplier is great - you can bring in your old containers for a refill if you like.

Whilst an organic aqueous cream is likely to cost a bit more, it can still prove more cost effective than buying a range of different treatment oils that may go off later. The one my supplier makes is a combination of Sweet Almond oil and Grape Seed oil.

If you really cannot find a supplier, or are keen on DIY creams, you can look up making your own base on the internet. It is quite a tricky process though and I have found that it is much simpler to buy it ready made. Still, if that is something that interests you, check around online - there are plenty of recipes available.

Whilst I prefer an organic base, I will use an everyday cream at a push. If expense is a problem for you, save the organic cream to use on your face and use the normal stuff on your body. It is not as nourishing but does still provide some moisture and the essential oils added do boost its effectiveness.

I prefer to use a cream base for making day treatments. For night treatments, I stick to cream in spring and summer and an oil base in fall and winter.

Get yourself a few glass jars that have lids that screw on tightly. A shorter jar with a wider mouth is a far better idea in this case - this allows you to scoop out the cream more easily.

It is also a good idea to buy some labels at the same time. I usually look for circular labels that I can put on the bottom of the bottle or the lid of the bottle so that they are less likely to be damaged by oil spilling. Alternatively, cover the labels with clear film and stick it down well. If they do get cream spilled on them, they will turn clear and you will not be able to read the writing on them.

Write your label out as you are making your blend so that you don't forget the ingredients - list the date, the oils used and what the blend is meant to treat. Do take this extra step or you risk ending up with a cupboard full of half-used bottles that you have forgotten the ingredients to.

Also, if a blend works well, you want to be able to duplicate it easily in future.

When it comes to the right dilution of essential oils to cream, it is actually pretty easy to work out - you will use no more than 6 drops of essential oils for each 10ml of cream and this dosage is only to be resorted to in severe cases.

You should only use half this maximum dose when creating a cream for your face as the skin on the face is a lot more delicate.

To be on the safe side, always start at a lower dosage of oils and always do a patch test first before applying them all over. If the oils do not irritate the skin, you may increase the concentration as long as it never exceeds 6 drops for every 10ml of cream.

If there is a reaction and you have used a blend of oils, you may need to test each oil individually to see which one is causing the adverse reaction.

When making your cream, it is important to stir the cream very well so that the oils are completely incorporated. I use a clean paddle stick to do this but a wooden skewer works just as well. If you are using your kitchen utensils, stick to stainless steel ones only - silicone and plastic will absorb the odors of the oils and become unsuitable for use in food preparation.

I normally only make up enough to last a couple of weeks or so so I don't usually worry about adding preservatives. To prevent bacterial growth in the cream, make sure that the jars are sterilized before use and always clean your hands thoroughly before applying the cream. If this is something that is of concern to you, you can add a capsule of Vitamin E oil for every 250ml of cream used. Vitamin E oil is a natural preservative.

Using a fixative oil like Sandalwood or Cedar Wood is also a good way to preserve the blend naturally.

That said, in twenty or so years I have relied on Sandalwood as a fixative and never really bothered with the Vitamin E. The only time I had a problem with a cream going off was when I added fresh plant matter to the cream - and it was only one out of three batches that went off in that case.

# Carrier Oils

In aromatherapy practice, it is more common to blend the oils into a carrier oil. This makes for a more deeply moisturizing treatment overall. If you do not like using oil on your skin, stick to the aqueous cream. It is a commonly held belief that using oil on your skin will cause it to become blocked and spotty but, if you use the right oil, this is a false belief. Grape Seed oil, for example, is a lighter and more toning oil that can help to balance excess sebum in the skin.

The general rule when it comes to choosing a carrier base for use on your skin is that the drier the skin is, the more nourishing the oil that is needed. Sweet Almond oil is a more nourishing oil and can be used on all skin types.

Boost the treatment value of your oil by adding in special treatment oils at a concentration of about 10%. You will often find that the richer oils like Avocado oil have a texture that is unpleasant to use neat on your skin.

If you need a quick massage base oil to use, you can turn to your kitchen cupboards. Sunflower oil does not have a pleasant texture but it is absorbed okay and is quite handy if you need to give someone a quick shoulder rub.

I used to have a very fine rash of bumps on my upper arms - the skin there was very dry and so I blended Olive oil with Neroli oil, Sandalwood oil and Geranium oil. I massaged in morning and evening and the bumps went away. A good quality olive oil is deeply moisturizing and also has anti-bacterial and anti-fungal properties.

I would advise against using either of these oils on the face as they are not refined enough - even when applied to the body there is usually some excess that needs to be wiped away. Here are some of the oils that you may consider instead:

## Sweet Almond Oil or Apricot Kernel Oil

These are both from the same family and tend to have similar properties. Both oil are rich in nutrients and suitable for use on all skin types. They are one of the richer oils and so suit those with dry or irritated skin well. They are very soothing to use and will not irritate sensitive skin. If you need to treat eczema, these are the ideal base oils. Use with care or avoid altogether if you have an allergy to nuts.

Sweet Almond oil contains Vitamins A, B1, B2 and B6. The oil does have a small amount of Vitamin E in it and it is a very stable oil to use. This oil lasts well and does not go rancid very quickly. You are typically looking at a shelf-life of around about a year to two years.

## Avocado Oil

You may have a choice between refined and unrefined Avocado oil as it is sold both ways. Stick to the refined varieties. Even these are very rich and feel quite heavy. It is said that Avocado oil mimics the skin's own oils almost exactly. Because of the density of the oil, it is better to use it in lower concentrations. If you have severely dry or damaged skin, mix equal quantities of Avocado oil and another oil. For normal day to day use, a 10% - 20% concentration of the oil is more than enough.

Because it has a similar structure to the skin's own, it is fairly easily absorbed. It makes a wonderful anti-aging treatment and is great for healing burned skin and scar tissue.

It contains Vitamins A, B1, B2 and D as well as Lecithin. It does not, unfortunately, keep very well so you should only buy smaller bottles. You are looking at a shelf life of around 6 months to a year in absolutely ideal conditions.

## Calendula Oil

Calendula oil is a nourishing oil and promotes skin regeneration. It will help acne heal and prevent further scarring. You can add it into your cream to help heal burns and stretchmarks. For a real boost, also add in Hypericum oil.

This oil is good to use on the face and will help to reduce the appearance of thread veins. It can also help to heal varicose veins. It makes a wonderful addition to a cream to moisturize and heal dry, irritated skin that is prone to rashes.

If you suffer with dry eczema, a 10% concentration of Calendula oil applied twice daily will work wonders.

Mix 3-6 drops of Chamomile oil and apply to your cheek over the site of a tooth extraction for pain relief.

This oil contains Vitamins A, B, D and E and is not likely to go rancid too quickly. You are looking at an average shelf life of between 1 and 2 years.

## Coconut Oil

Coconut oil became the darling of the health industry a few years ago but it has long been used in beauty treatments to moisturize hair and skin. The oil is solid at room temperature and so makes an excellent base for lip balms and body butters. If you want a more liquid texture, you will need to heat the oil and add equal quantities of another carrier oil.

Coconut oil is absorbed well by the skin and makes it silky smooth and soft. It is a rich oil that can be used on any different skin type. That said, it is known to cause skin rashes so it should be used more sparingly. It is better to get the cold-pressed oil as there is less chance of solvent residue in it.

The oil contains Trimyristin, Caproic Acids and Glycerides and is a very stable oil, even at higher temperatures. You are looking at a shelf-life of 1 - 2 years.

## Evening Primrose Oil

This is an oil that contains a high proportion of healing fatty acids and is suitable for use on all skin types. It is especially useful to those with skin that is on the dry and irritated side and it makes a good anti-aging treatment as well. It is often used in blends to treat psoriasis and eczema and is an excellent oil to use to help heal wounds. It can help reduce scarring.

Only Borage oil has a higher concentration of gamma linoleic acid. It also contains oleic acid and linoleic acid in significant quantities as well. This oil lasts well - you have a shelf-life of around 1 - 2 years.

## Grape Seed Oil

Sweet Almond oil and Grape Seed oil are the top two choices for aromatherapists because they are very stable oils, have a long shelf life and are well-absorbed by the body.

Grape Seed oil can be used by people with any skin type but benefits those with skins that are oilier and those that have larger pores. The oil is a little lighter than Sweet Almond oil and more astringent.

If you are using Grape Seed oil, make sure that it is the refined variety - the unrefined variety is less expensive but is not recommended for therapeutic use at all.

Grape Seed oil contains Vitamin E and Linoleic acid and lasts very well. It has a shelf-life of around 1 - 2 years.

## Hazelnut Oil

This oil is an astringent oil and is suitable for use on oily or combination skin. It is a little too harsh for dry, sensitive skin. It is great for treating acne though. Check whether you are getting pure Hazelnut oil - it is one of the more expensive oils and is often diluted with other oils.

It contains Oleic acid and Linoleic acid and lasts relatively well. It has a shelf-life or around 1 - 1 ½ years.

## Jojoba Oil/ Wax

Jojoba is a very popular component of many commercial skin preparations. It is extremely nourishing but does not clog up the pores of the skin. It can help acne to heal and reduce the inflammation present. It reduces scarring.

What is not as well known is that Jojoba is useful in helping reduce inflammation associated with rheumatism and arthritis.

It is more of a wax than an oil as it remains solid at room temperature. If you need a more viscous oil, mix it with equal quantities of a different carrier oil.

It has a large proportion of Vitamin E making it less prone to oxidation. It will last well and you may add it into a blend to help extend the shelf-life of the blend as a whole. It has a shelf-life of around 2 years.

# Macadamia Nut

Macadamia Nut oil is one of the best oils for anti-aging. It is suitable for use on any skin type but is particularly helpful to dry, mature skin. Apply daily before going out to boost your skin's natural protection against the sun. It helps restore normal sebum production and is very similar in makeup to the skin's own sebum.

It contains oleic acid and palmitoleic acid. It does not oxidize easily and can be used to extend the shelf-life of any blend. It has a shelf-life or around 2 years.

# Wheatgerm Oil

This is a really great oil for anti-aging as it has a high anti-oxidant content. It is best to use it in smaller concentrations - no more than 5% - 10% at a time. The texture and the scent of the oil at higher concentrations can be off-putting.

It is very nourishing for dry and mature skin and helps damaged skin to regenerate. It can assist in clearing up allergic skin reactions.

What is not as well known is that it is also great for loosening up stiff and sore muscles.

If applying to the face, use it no more than twice a week as it can stimulate hair production.

It has high levels of Vitamin E, phytosterols, Vitamin A, Vitamin B Complex and lecithin. It lasts very well due to its high anti-oxidant content and can help to extend the shelf-life of other blends. It has a shelf-life of around 2 years.

# Special Treatment Oils

The following oils can be added in need when the skin is in need of a little bit of extra care and a boost. With these oils it is generally better to keep to about 10% concentration and to blend with either Sweet Almond oil or Grape Seed oil.

## Borage Oil

Borage oil is highly nourishing and can help to soothe irritated skin. It can be added in very low concentrations to a treat eczema and psoriasis. Use the oil at a maximum concentration of 10%.

## Carrot Oil

Can sooth and calm irritated skin.

## Castor Oil

Whilst this is quite commonly found in cosmetics, I find that it has a rather unpleasant texture and is quite sticky. That said, if you have an abscess or sore, it can help to fight off infection and help the wound to heal. Apply neat to the area that requires treatment. If you would like to try it in a blend for moisturizing, add no more than 5% concentration. Frankly though, there are much better oils for moisturizing.

## Cocoa Butter

This is a nice moisturizing oil but I usually add it in more for the aroma then anything else. If you are on a tight budget, this is not an essential treatment oil.

# Lime Blossom Oil

This is a great oil to have on hand. It can help to reduce the appearance of wrinkles, is soothing and relaxing if you have trouble sleeping and can help to relieve pain and swelling if you are arthritic.

# Linseed Oil

This has a high proportion of fatty acids and is a great healer and soother. Use in lower concentrations - no more than 10%.

# Meadowsweet Oil

If you battle with arthritic or rheumatic pain, this is a good oil to get. Massage in twice daily to help reduce swelling and provide pain relief.

# Palm Kernel Oil

This is similar to coconut oil in terms of properties and less likely to cause skin reactions. The actual color of the oil can be a little off-putting and I would advise using a lower concentration of between 5% and 10%.

# Peanut Oil

Peanut oil has strong anti-inflammatory properties and can help reduce arthritic pain.

# Rosehip Oil

This is one of the best anti-aging treatments and can be used neat on the skin. It has high levels of Vitamin C in it and helps the skin to regenerate. Apply after cleansing the skin and allow to soak in for a few minutes before wiping off residue.

## St John's Wort/Hypericum

If you have burnt skin, this is a good oil to have on hand. Mix one part Hypericum oil and one part Calendula oil, add in a drop or two of Geranium oil and a drop of Lavender oil and a drop of Palmrosa oil and the skin will heal much faster.

# Chapter 10: Hairapy with Essential Oils

## Say Goodbye to Those Bad Hair Days Forever

We all know that we should eat well and avoid over-styling our hair to keep it in tip-top shape. That is something that we know but it is not always something that we follow through on.

Fortunately, essential oils can go a long way to helping nourish the hair and conditioning the scalp. Rosemary oil, West Indian Bay oil and Clary Sage oil are all great to help bring an oily scalp back into balance and kill off any bacteria. Use diluted in oil and rub into the scalp. Rosemary can stimulate new hair growth and help to condition hair. Used in a rinse, it can help to maintain the color of dark hair. Use Chamomile oils in a rinse for light hair to help it shine.

Lavender oil helps to untangle hair when used in the rinse water and, when rubbed into the scalp, helps to condition it.

You can add a coupe of drops of Lavender or Rosemary oils to your shampoo or conditioner to easily incorporate them into your hair care routine.

Oil treatments are the best conditioners for hair - even if you have greasy hair, you should use an oil treatment once a week. In most cases, you will warm up the oil a little, add your chosen essential oils and then rub the oil into the scalp - If you have greasy hair, stop here. If your hair is dry or frazzled, massage the mixture through to the end of the hair shaft. Wrap your hair and scalp in cling film and a warm towel to really intensify the treatment and leave on for at least 20 minutes.

When you are ready to wash the oil out of the hair, you do not wash your hair as normal. Instead of wetting your hair first and then applying the shampoo, you will mix the shampoo into a handful of water and then massage that into the scalp and ends of the hair. Rinse and repeat and the oil should be gone.

## Amla Oil

If you can get hold of Amla oil, also known as Indian Gooseberry oil, you can use it as carrier oil for your other oils. The trick with Amla oil is to only rub it into your scalp - do not massage into the shaft of the hair itself as this can leave the hair feeling dry. Rub into the scalp and leave on overnight. When you rinse it off the next morning, you will be amazed at how soft and manageable your hair becomes.

## Warming Oil For Hair Treatments

All you need to do is to measure out the oil that you are going to use and put it into a wide-mouthed jar. Boil the kettle and find a bowl that the jar fits into and stand the jar in it. When the kettle has boiled, pour boiling water into the bowl so that it surrounds the jar of oil and reaches about half-way up the jar. Let the oil stand for about 10 minutes to warm nicely.

Alternatively you can warm the oil in the microwave but do be careful doing this or you could make it too hot. Warm for a minute on a lower setting - you want the oil to be at skin temperature when you use it, not scalding.

In either case, add the essential oils just before you apply the treatment.

## The Ultimate Hair Conditioner for Oily Hair

This helps to condition the hair and to stimulate growth.

25ml Olive oil, slightly warmed.

5 Drops Rosemary oil

5 Drops Lavender oil

Warm the oil using the method mentioned above. Add the oils. Apply to the scalp, massaging in. Wrap your head in cling wrap and a warm towel. Leave on for 20 minutes before rinsing out.

## The Ultimate Hair Conditioner for Dry Hair

25ml Jojoba oil, slightly warmed

5 Drops Vertiver oil

5 Drops Lavender oil

Warm the oil using the method mentioned above. Add the oils. Apply to the scalp, massaging in. Wrap your head in cling wrap and a warm towel. Leave on for 20 minutes before rinsing out.

## On the Go Scalp Rub

5 Drops Lavender oil

5 Drops Tea Tree oil

Massage the oils into your scalp and carry on with your day. You do not need to rinse them out of your hair.

# Hair Tonic

10 Drops Rosemary/ Chamomile oils (Depending on whether your hair is dry or not)

1 Tablespoon of Apple Cider Vinegar

100ml Lavender or Rose Water

Mix the ingredients together well and then massage into the scalp. Leave on for at least half an hour or overnight. If you can get away with it, do not rinse out until the next time you need to wash your hair, the longer it stays on, the better.

# Dry Shampoo

1 Drop Rosemary oil

1 Tablespoon Fuller's Earth or Powdered Orris Root

Mix the powder and the Rosemary oil together and apply to the greasy parts of your head. Leave in place for about 5 minutes so that excess oil can be absorbed.

# Chapter 11: Beautiful You With Essential Oils

## Enhancing Your Own Beauty Naturally

Aging in our family has never really been a huge issue - both the men and women in our family age well. That said there is a also a lot to be said for looking after your skin and as kids this was something that my grandmother consistently drummed into me.

Admittedly, I stick to simpler blends and creams and I do fall off the rails every now and again. Still, even though I have been less than dedicated when it comes to skin care, my skin is still aging very well. I attribute this to using the natural creams that my grandmother taught me to make.

I also have a skin that burns easily and so steer clear of the sun as much as possible and that also probably helps.

It is quite amazing to me how effective natural treatments can be - there is really no need to spend hundreds of dollars a year on expensive creams that simply don't compete.

Essential oils are completely natural and easily absorbed and used by the skin. As you start to get older, your skin begins to lose elasticity and becomes far more dehydrated. Fine lines and wrinkles start to develop.

Luckily, it is never too late to start improving the skin.

# Moisture Please

Skin that is improperly hydrated will always have problems - either the sebum production gets pushed into overdrive causing spots and oily skin or the skin becomes dry and tight.

# Simplify Please

Starting today, you need to start concentrating as much on what goes onto your skin as you do on what goes into your mouth. Quality, natural essential oil based creams and oils have the ingredients that your skin needs without a lot of artificial chemicals and fillers.

I remember many, many years ago when the first Alpha-Hydroxy-Acid products came out onto the market. My friend tried one and found that it was too harsh for her skin. She went back to the counter and mentioned this and was made to feel small because there was no way, according to the consultant, that that product would cause a reaction.

The reason that I have never forgotten this is that same company brought out a milder product within a year as it became obvious that the AHA's should be available at different dilutions.

The problem with the beauty industry today is that everyone is looking for the next big thing when it comes to anti-aging. Millions is spent on research and advertising to convince you that their products are the best.

With such a rush to get to the latest new thing, who's to say these products are actually worth the amounts you spend on them and who's to say that they actually work anyway?

Essential oils are a constant - the haven't changed a whole lot and are very effective. Simplify your life - you really only need a cleanser, possibly a toner, a day cream and a night cream. I would buy a commercial eye cream simply because it really is not a good idea to get the oils too close to the eyes - this can cause to a build-up of product under the eye and a puffy look. If you do want to go natural here as well, you can dab in small amounts of plain Rose Hip oil.

You can supplement your regimen with scrubs and face marks a couple of times a week. Aside from that, you really need little else.

If you do wear make-up, a cotton ball dipped in Sweet Almond or Grape Seed oil will clear it away. Any excess left over can be removed by wiping face with a clean wash cloth that has been soaked in warm water. You can, if you want to, lay the warm cloth over the skin for a few minutes just so that the pores open and any remaining dirt comes to the surface. Rinse cloth and wipe again.

Toning the skin is easily accomplished using natural treatments. A hydro-sol can be a great way to tone the skin. The hydro sol is the water that remains over after the essential oils have been extracted. It still retains some of the essence of the oil.

Alternatively look for Witch Hazel if you have a greasy skin or Rose Water or Orange Blossom Water if you have a drier skin to tone the skin.

Now you either apply the night cream or the day cream. Your night cream is where you can add your special treatment products without needing to worry whether or not the oils are photo-toxic, i.e. they react to the sun and this can cause skin sensitization or discoloration.

Once a week, apply your scrub - keep it gentle so that you can apply your face mask directly afterwards. I know that most magazines will advise against doing a scrub and a face mask on the same day but I disagree with this sentiment.

As long as you use a gentle scrub, you run no risk of damaging the skin and the deep cleanse of the scrub actually increases the efficiency of the face mask overall.

Now onto the recipes!

## Night Time Healer

This oils is very nourishing and will boost moisture and reduce the appearance of fine lines and wrinkles and help to reverse sun damage and scarring.

100ml Rose Hip oil

10ml Avocado oil

5 drops Sandalwood oil

5 drops Geranium oil

5 drops Neroli oil

5 drops Rose oil

5 drops Lavender oil

Clean and tone face as outlined above. Using 1 finger, apply a dot about the size of your finger pad to each cheek and dab in - do no rub as this pulls the skin and can create lines.

Use another two of these drops to cover your forehead and temples. One more dot should be enough to cover the T-Zone. You'll need about three dots for the neck and about four for the decolletage. Finish off by dotting one dot onto the back of each hand and massaging in.

Relax for 5-10 minutes, placing a warmed wash cloth - damp not soaking - over the face to further assist the absorption of the oils. Dab off any excess after this time and dab skin dry.

This starts working to clarify and moisturize your skin from the very first treatment.

From the first application, you will notice that your face glows after this treatment.

## Day to Day Cream

Naturally, you want different things from your night and day cream.

80 ml aqueous cream, preferably organic

10 drops palmarosa oil

5 drops geranium oil

5 drops sandalwood oil

Cleanse and tone skin and apply. Go off to style your hair or start breakfast so that the cream is completely absorbed before applying your make up.

These two simple creams will help heal your skin and it will soon start to look younger and more refined. The day cream is mild enough to be used by people of all skin types because Geranium oil is a skin regulator - it helps to moisturize dry skin and helps to regulate sebum production thus curbing acne as well.

# Easy Face Scrub

1 Wash cloth, clean

½ Cup of oatmeal

2 drops Lavender oil

2 drops Tea Tree oil (If you have oily skin)

Place the oatmeal in the center of the cloth and ball it up. Soak in warm water for a couple of minutes and then gently massage over the skin. The wash cloth should only be used for this purpose and should never be softened. That way, it will provide a good, gentle scrubbing surface.

The oatmeal inside will also help to intensify the cleansing action but will release a liquid that is highly moisturizing.

# Honey Face Mask

10 ml Avocado oil/ a half a mashed up avocado

10ml Sweet almond oil

2 Tablespoons honey

Mix together all ingredients and apply to face. This is a very moisturizing treatment and well worth a bit of mess. Leave on for 20-30 minutes and then cleanse face as normal.

Give yourself a soothing deep moisturizing treatment once a week by mashing up half an avocado, mixed with 2 tablespoons of honey, and applying it as a mask to your skin.

Don't waste fruit peels either when it comes to natural treatments. Papaya makes a great nourishing treatment that refines pores and is slightly astringent. Eat your papaya, rub the skin onto your cleansed face. Leave for about 5 minutes before washing off again.

# Flower Waters

It is possible to make toilet or flower water at home by adding about 20 to 30 drops of essential oil to a 100ml bottle of spring or de-ionized water, leaving it for a few days in the dark and then filtering it using a coffee filter paper. Although essential oils do not dissolve in water they do impart their scent to it as well as their properties.

This method can be very helpful in the prevention and treatment of skin conditions such as acne, dermatitis and eczema, and to generally tone and cleanse the complexion. Almost any oil can be used, but the more traditional ones include rose, orange blossom, lavender and petitgrain; alternatively, blended flower waters can be made to suit specific complexions.

Orange Blossom water is probably the most famous skin treatment of all and was, according to legend, first used by the then Queen of Hungary to keep her young and beautiful.

# Using Milk as a Treatment

The lactic acid in milk acts to gently exfoliate the skin and to improve it's ability to retain moisture. You can either add it to your bath water or use it as a facial cleanser - it is especially good for those with blemishes or greasy skin.

If using it in the bath, ½ to 1 cup of full-fat milk is best. If using as a cleanser, make only enough to last the day and add 2-3 drops of your chosen essential oil for every 5 teaspoons of milk.

Goat's milk is preferable to cow's milk, especially in the cases where skin allergies and eczema are present.

## Make Your Own Talcum Powder

Using rice flour, you can make your own fine talcum powder and not have to worry about synthetic scents and other ingredients that might irritate your skin.

This is another great way to incorporate essential oils into your daily life. Make a powder to match your scent so that you can layer it.

Mix in 3-5 drops of essential oils for every 2 tablespoons of rice flower. Store in an airtight container and use as required.

## Witch Hazel as a Toner

Witch Hazel makes a very effective toner for those with oily skins and acne and can help to unclog pores and reduce their appearance. You can add 2 drops of Tea Tree oil and 2 Drops of Lavender oil into 100ml of Witch Hazel and use as a spot treatment.

Neat Witch Hazel is too harsh for dry and sensitive skin so either mix in equal parts of Witch Hazel and Rose Water or Orange Blossom water or steer clear of the Witch Hazel completely.

## The Best Oils for Skin Care

For skin regeneration you cannot beat Lavender oil, Chamomile oil, Rose oil, Neroli oil, Frankincense oil, Palmrosa oil and Geranium oil.

For dry skin use: Lavender oil, Chamomile oil, Rose oil, Neroli oil, Frankincense oil, Geranium oil or Sandalwood oil.

For oily skin use: Lavender oil, Tea Tree oil, Geranium oil, Juniper Berry oil, Lemon oil or Rosemary oil.

# Chapter 12:  Healthy You With Essential Oils

## Enhancing Your Health Naturally

Once you start to use essential oils, you are bound to become more in tune with your body's own signs and rhythms and will be able to predict with greater accuracy when a headache will strike, for example.

This is a really important thing when it comes to improving your health. If you can get a Migraine off track as soon as it begins to develop, by massaging in a Lavender and Chamomile blend into your neck, you will not only reduce the severity but also the chances that it will move into a full-blown attack. You might even head it off completely.

Pretty soon, you will become in tune with the early signs if illness and will be able to treat them accordingly.

There is no time like the present so why not start the next time you have a stuffy nose? Having a cold or flu can be awful - your sinuses ache, your head aches and your whole body feels sore and tired. It is not easy to get rid of a sinus headache either.

By choosing three simple oils, you can clear congestion and the headache quite quickly. Some blends that you get for colds and flu or headaches come in a glass container with a roller ball head - don't toss these out when the oils inside are finished. Rinse them out and add your own blend.

These sticks allow you to place targeted bursts of essential oils. In the case of a sinus headache, for example, you can roll the ball over just the sinuses to clear congestion.

If you have a sinus headache, or any other headache, you will notice that areas on your scalp become sore and tender. Also rub the stick over these areas. The combination of the oil and the pressure is often enough to help ease that headache.

If you don't have one of these stick applicators, simply apply the oils with your fingers and massage well into the scalp.

# Dealing With Chronic Pain

The sad fact is that most people deal with pain or illness in some form or another just about every day of their lives. In some cases, the pain is so severe that medication is abused and a tolerance develops leaving fewer and fewer opportunities to find relief.

Fortunately, essential oils can provide significant pain relief. For chronic conditions such as rheumatism, essential oils such as Sweet Marjoram, Melissa, Black Pepper, Eucalyptus, etc. can provide lasting relief.

The idea is to use the treatment as soon as the twinges start. If you want to, you may use the treatments as a  prophylactic measure, but should always switch the oils completely after three weeks and use a different set completely for the next three weeks.

## Super Pain Reliever

2 Drops Melissa oil

2 Drops Sweet Marjoram oil

2 Drops Chamomile oil

10ml Carrier oil of your choice

10ml Jojoba oil

Blend all ingredients together and massage into affected areas twice daily or as needed.

You can also cut out the carrier oil and Jojoba oil and use these oils in a hot bath instead. If you are not epileptic and do not have high blood pressure, you can also add 2 cups of Epsom Salts to the bath to help relieve pain.

## Boost Immunity

Once you have started dealing with how to treat illnesses as they arise, you can start to work on building your immunity to disease. All essential oils benefit immunity to some degree but the best for this are Tea Tree and Eucalyptus oil.

It isn't even very hard - all you need to do is to expose yourself to one or the other of these oils every day for about an hour. Repeat daily for three weeks and then switch to a different oil to prevent a tolerance developing.

Pretty soon, you will find that you get ill less often and you will find that if you do get sick, it is with milder symptoms and a shorter duration.

# Chapter 13: Happy You With Essential Oils

## Improving Your Mood Naturally

Using oils that you love the smell of and that have good associations for you on a day to day basis will help to improve your mood. When testing oils or blends, it is a good idea to analyze how they effect you emotionally as well checking what the benefits to using them are.

Ideally speaking, find a few different oils that make you feel happier and brighter - Bergamot, Neroli, Rose and Jasmine are just three examples of such oils. Now start using them in your day to day life.

This could be as simple as diffusing the oils. If you are in an office environment and this is not allowed, there are a couple of things that you an do - make a basic hand cream using the essential oil blends of choice. (Just be careful not to use photo-toxic oils if you are going out into the sun.)

Alternatively you can carry a handkerchief sprinkled with the oils and inhale them every now and again. The oils won't last all day so you will need to add more oils.

The simplest alternative by far is to get hold of an opaque plastic or glass bottle with a tight-fitting lid. Either place some tissues or some cotton wool into the bottle, sprinkle on two or three drops of essential oil and seal. Every time you open the bottle, you will get that wonderful, uplifting scent coming out at you.

Keep the bottle in your office drawer or, at a push, your car. That way when you are having a really bad day at work there is a remedy close to hand.

The bottle prevents the essential oils from evaporating too quickly and so you only need to top up the oils once every one or two months.

A great alternative is a roller stick. You may have to buy one with oils in already as these are not that easy to get unused if you are only buying one or two bottles. Once the oils have been finished, lever out the ball section of the lid, rinse well and add your own carrier oils and essential oils.

Making yourself happier through essential oils is quite easy - start incorporating the oils that make you feel good into your personal skin care routine, into your final rinse water when doing washing, etc.

Switch out the oils every once in a while so that you do not develop a tolerance for them.

## Happy Day Blend

2 Drops Jasmine oil

2 Drops Benzoin oil

2 Drops Neroli oil

Mix oils together and diffuse them in whatever way seems best to you. Allow at least one hour of exposure a day for a week to see really good results.

# Frazzled Nerve Blend

2 Drops Frankincense oil

2 Drops Sandalwood oil

2 Drops Neroli oil

Blend all the oils together and diffuse them for at least 1 hour to get ultimate results. This blend is extremely relaxing and so is good to use during the evening. It is also a good blend to use if you want to meditate.

# Come On Get Happy Blend

2 Drops Bergamot oil

2 Drops Jasmine oil

2 Drops Neroli oil

2 Drops Sandalwood oil

Mix oils together and diffuse them in whatever way seems best to you. Allow at least one hour of exposure a day for a week to see really good results.

If it more that you are fatigued rather than actually depressed, you can start using essential oils that stimulate the mind and senses to help you make it though each day.

Fresh smelling oils such as Camphor, Rosemary, Basil, Peppermint and Eucalyptus can help you to shake off fatigue and allow you to get through the day at work.

Once you are home, make sure that there is a cut-off point when work stops completely. After this point there is no checking business emails, writing reports, etc.

Start winding down for bed at least an hour before you want to sleep. Switch off the TV , smart phone and computer and choose relaxing oils such as Chamomile, Vetiver, Sandalwood and Melissa. Diffuse a relaxing blend for about an hour before bedtime to help you sleep really, really well. Spend the time doing something relaxing like reading or knitting and put a nice relaxing CD on to play.

Mix feel-good oils into your hand lotion and make a point of rubbing them into your hands, forearms and elbows every evening - your skin will start to look better and you will feel better as well.

Essential oils that are good for dealing with depression and a low mood include Benzoin, Neroli oil, Bergamot oil, Chamomile oil.

Need to put a bit of a spark back in the sex life? The following oils will help with this goal: Black pepper oil, Cardamon oil, Clary Sage oil, Neroli oi, Jasmine oil, Rose oil, Sandalwood oil, Patchouli oil and Ylang Ylang oil.

Oils to help you sleep include: Chamomile oil, Bergamot, Sandalwood oil, Lavender oil, Sweet Marjoram oil, Lemon Balm oil, Hops oil, Valerian oil, Lemon oil.

Oils that can help you recover from periods of stress and nervous fatigue include, Basil oil, Jasmine oil, Peppermint oil, Ylang Ylang oil, Neroli oil, Angelica oil, Rosemary oil.

Oils that support the nervous system include Chamomile oil, Clary Sage oil, Juniper oil, Lavender oil, Sweet Marjoram oil, Rosemary oil.

# Chapter 14: Baby, You and Essential Oils

## Aromatherapy and New Mothers

You can use some essential oils when you are pregnant but you do need to be very careful which oils you choose. An oil such as Rosemary oil, for example, can stimulate the uterus and cause an abortion of the foetus.

If you are trying to fall pregnant or are in your first trimester, I would advise using only the very gentlest of oils - Lavender and Chamomile,unless under the recommendation of a licensed aromatherapist.

Check out any oils that you may like to use and if you do not feel comfortable that it may be safe, leave it out completely.

## NEVER Use These Oils if You Are Pregnant

These are dangerous for the baby as they may cause uterine contractions. If you are trying to have a child, think there is a possibility that you are pregnant or have been diagnosed as pregnant don't even think about using these oils:

Basil oil, Clove oil, Cinnamon oil, Myrrh oil, Rosemary oil, Sage oil, Thyme oil. These oils can cause a miscarriage.

# In Your Final Trimester

You may add these oils in low concentrations in your final trimester:

Fennel oil, Rose oil, Peppermint oil, Cedar Wood oil.

Again, if you are unsure, just rather leave the oil out altogether.

## Stop Stretchmarks From Developing

*Carrier Oils:*

15ml of Borage oil

15ml of Rose-Hip oil

60ml of Jojoba oil

*Essential Oils*:

4 Drops Neroli oil

4 Drops Frankincense oil

2 Drops Lavender oil

Mix everything together - any of the essential oils can be exchanged for the others though this blend is particularly effective at reducing the formation and appearance of stretch marks. If you cannot find the Borage oil, substitute with either Rose-Hip or Jojoba oils.

Once you have passed the first trimester, you can also add in 2 drops of Geranium oil to boost this blend even more.

This is also a mix that can help lift your spirits and help you to relax.

Massage gently into the tummy and breast area at least twice a day.

# A Less Sweet Blend

*Carrier Oils:*

15ml of Borage oil

15ml of Rose-Hip oil

60ml of Jojoba oil

*Essential Oils:*

4 Drops Vetiver oil

4 Drops Sandalwood oil

2 Drops Lavender oil

Also use twice a day. This blend is also great for helping you to relax and will help soothed frayed nerves and sore muscles.

## Reducing Anxiety and Depression During Pregnancy

Pregnancy is supposed to be the happiest time of your life but the truth is that it doesn't always feel that way. With hormones in the body raging, your mood can swing from angel to Queen of Evil in a matter of minutes. I once worked with a woman who really battled with pregnancy - she apologized ahead of time because pregnancy turned her into a real witch. Whilst this is an extreme example, having a blend of oils on hand can help to boost mood and help you to feel a little better.

Worries about the change in your body size and shape can be allayed a little by massaging soothing oils into the skin so that at least you need not worry as much about getting stretchmarks.

Get your partner in on the action and have them run you a nice warm bath. Add in 2 drops of Neroli oil, 2 Drops of Lavender oil and 2 Drops of Sandalwood oil and feel the anxiety and aches soak away.

Alternatively, blend the same oils into 100ml of Sweet Almond oil and let your partner give you a nice, relaxing shoulder rub.

Vetiver oil is another deeply relaxing essential oil and can re-balance the emotions and stave off stress. Vetiver smells rich and earthy and can be used on its own or in a blend to great success.

## Reducing Aches During Pregnancy

As baby grows, he becomes heavier and heavier and your own body starts to ache more and more. Since the Ibuprofen is off the menu, you might want to try some essential oils to help you feel better.

The good news is that Chamomile essential oil is the most effective of all the oils when it comes to pain relief and reducing inflammation an it is gentle enough to be used throughout your pregnancy without fear of complications. Blending it with Lavender oil makes it a highly effective pain killer, a good treatment for skin and a soothing blend for the nerves that will help you sleep better at night.

## Sweet Chamomile Blend

*Carrier Oils:*

20ml Sweet Almond oil

*Essential Oils:*

3 drops Lavender oil

3 Drops Chamomile oil

Rub into you back or whatever part of your body is aching at least once or twice a day. I often find it useful to follow up the application of the oil with a warm shower. Give the oil about 10 minutes to be absorbed and then have a warm shower. The heat from the shower will help any leftovers sink in and will also help to enhance the relaxing effects of the treatment.

## Oil To Help Muscle Aches After the First Trimester

*Carrier Oils:*

20ml Sweet Almond oil

*Essential Oils:*

3 drops Vetiver oil

3 Drops Geranium oil

3 Drops Sandalwood oil

Rub into the area at least once or twice a day.

## Cold Compress for Relief from Heat and Headaches

If are your biggest in the heat of summer there is good news and bad news - the good news is that you won't be getting up in the freezing cold for nightly feeds. The bad news is that so close to the end of your pregnancy, the hot weather can really make you uncomfortable.

Cool compresses form a double function - they help to physically cool you down and act as a delivery system for the essential oils that you want to use.

You'll need a wash cloth and a bowl of cool water. You add the essential oils to the water and less the wash cloth soak in it. The wash cloth is then wrung out and placed on the back of the neck or on your forehead to help you cool down.

What I sometimes do is to use two wash cloths, soaking the second one while the first is in use. Swap the clothes out when the first has warmed up.

Add the following oils:

2 Drops of Lavender oil

2 Drops of Chamomile oil

1 Drop of Sandalwood oil

1 Drop of Neroli (Optional)

# Enjoy Your Pregnancy

If you find that you are prone to blue moods, grab a bottle of neroli oil and sprinkle a few drops onto a handkerchief or tissue. Sniff repeatedly through the day - keep on hand so that you can get to it easily. My mother told me about this one and she used to stick the tissue in the sleeve of her jersey to keep it easily accessible.

A drop or two of Sandalwood oil will help to reduce feelings of anxiety.

If you are finding that it is tough to cope or feel overwhelmed, also add a drops of Chamomile oil.

If these oils do not appeal to you, Vetiver is a good option from the second trimester onwards - it is relaxing and grounding and not as sweet as the floral oils.

Once you know what oils are safe to use, feel free to experiment a bit. Due to the hormonal changes, a blend that you find wonderful today could leaving you feeling nauseous in a week's time so it is good to have some backups just in case.

# Beating Post-Natal Depression

Post-Natal Depression seems so unnatural - how can we be depressed after bringing a new life into the world? It can also make new mothers feel that something is wrong with them. If you consider that a baby means a big life change and that you are sleep deprived as well, it is actually a wonder that more people don't suffer from post-natal depression.

There is nothing wrong with basic post-natal depression, but if you feel as though you are totally overwhelmed or if you feel that you will hurt your child, it is important to get help. The real you would never in a million years do anything to harm your baby but post-natal depression can take on a more sinister side so get help if you need it and don't feel alone - it happens to a lot of new mothers.

2 Drops Neroli oil

2 Drops Lavender oil

2 Drops Ylang Ylang oil

2 Drops Sandalwood oil

Use this in a burner, or add to 20ml of a carrier oil of your choice and massage into skin.

Alternatively, this blend can really help to lift depression:

2 Drops Neroli oil

2 Drops Benzoin oil

2 Drops Cedarwood oil

Use this in a burner, or add to 20ml of a carrier oil of your choice and massage into skin. Alternatively, add it to you bath water.

# Essential Oils and Your Kids

Essential oils can be used for your kids but here you again need to do a little research. Not all oils are suitable to use on kids and you must use the oils that you can use in much lower dilutions than you would on yourself.

It must be remembered that the smaller your child is, the lower the dosage of essential oils must be. Would you, for example, give your baby the same dose of cold medication that your would take? Of course not! The same rule applies to essential oil usage.

Start out by doing a patch test on your skin to make sure that your skin is not irritated by the oil. If your skin tingles, reduce the concentration and repeat until a suitable concentration is reached.

Also do a patch test on your child before dousing them in the oil to make sure that they are not allergic to it at all.

Start with the lowest possible concentration and increase only as necessary. NEVER exceed the maximum doses outlined below unless upon the recommendation of a licenced aromatherapist.

**0- 10 weeks**: For the first 10 weeks of his life, baby has enough to contend with and should not be exposed to essential oils. His system at this stage is not strong enough to properly process and excrete the oils and sensitization and toxic buildup could result.

**10 weeks - 1 year**: No more than 1 drop of essential oil in every 10ml of carrier oil.

**1 year -8 years**: No more than 2 drops of essential oil in every 10 ml of carrier oil.

Massage for babies can be a relaxing experience for mother and child. You should not massage baby if they are ill, have just been immunized, have just eaten or are about to eat. Always avoid areas where the skin is broken or where there is new scar tissue.

Always set up in a room that is warm enough for baby and proceed slowly, working your way up from the feet and gently working towards the heart. Use gentle strokes and make sure that baby is enjoying the process. Tug gently to loosen the limbs. Follow off with by wrapping baby in a nice cuddly towel or blanket and have a cuddle. Depending on the oils that you used, this should soon put baby to sleep.

## Blend for Skin Conditions in Young Children

1 Drop Chamomile oil

1 Drop Lavender oil

Mix into 20ml of sweet almond oil or a blend of sweet almond and avocado oils (10ml each.) Massage over the whole body, avoiding the genitals.

This blend can also help baby sleep.

## Blend for Colic in Young Children

1 Drop Mandarin oil or 1 Drop Sweet Orange oil and 1 drop of Lavender oil, mixed into 20ml of a carrier oil of your choice and massaged into the back, chest and abdomen twice a day.

# Dealing with Colds and Flu in Young Children

1 Drop Tea Tree oil, 1 Drop Eucalyptus oil and 1 drop of mixed into 30ml of the carrier oil of your choice or placed in a diffuser will help clear up symptoms of colds and flu.

# Chapter 15: Healthy Home with Essential Oils

## Beating Germs and Bad Smells Naturally

## The Best Oils for Home Cleaning

Add up to 8 drops of oils per small pail of tepid water. Soak your cleaning cloth in it, wring out and use. I advise against using the mixture on chopping boards though as residues might build up on these and get transferred to your food.

For toilets, add three drops of oil to the bowl, leave on overnight and then flush away in the morning.

For scenting clothes and linen, add 3-4 drops to your washing machine's final cycle.

**For kitchen/ bathroom surfaces:** Geranium oil and Lemon oil.

**For sanitizing the toilet:** Tea tree oil or Pine.

**To clean the tub or sinks:** Lavender oil and Grapefruit oil.

**For scenting laundry:** Lavender oil.

With your essential oils, some white spirit vinegar and some baking soda, you should be all set to throw out those commercial cleaners and start enjoying a home that is clean, sanitized and chemical free.

# Room Spritz

2 Drops of Lavender oil

2 Drops of Sandalwood oil

100ml Vodka (optional but fixes the scent)

400ml Water

1 Atomizer bottle

Mix up all the ingredients in the bottle and spray to freshen the room as necessary. The Vodka has no noticeable scent in the mix but helps to fix the scent of the oils and also helps to diffuse the oils in the water mix. (Oils won't mix with water but they will mix into the Vodka).

# Carpet Freshener

2 Drops Lavender oil

2 Drops Sandalwood oil

1 Cup baking soda

Mix the oils into the baking soda and make sure that they are well incorporated. Sprinkle the baking soda over your carpets and leave for a minimum of an hour, preferably overnight. Vacuum up and your carpets are lightly scented and much fresher smelling.

## Scented Drawer Liners

Making your own drawer liners is really simple - you can even recycle the Christmas wrapping paper that you were given. Alternatively, choose a pretty piece of wrapping paper or even some plain paper. All you need to do is to cut to the size of your drawers and place down flat in them. Sprinkle a few drops of essential oils over the paper and you are ready to go.

# Chapter 16: Happy Home Life With Essential Oils

## Create Harmony in the Home

Families are wonderful things - they support you in times of need and are there to help you celebrate the good times. Each family member has their own personality and this is usually a great thing. When you are living in close quarters though, upsets are bound to occur.

Essential oils can help to create a calmer feeling in the home in general. Diffusing Sandalwood oil, for example, can help everyone to feel calmer and it is usually a scent that is appreciated in the home.

## Choose Scent According to Mood

What is going on in the home when you want to use your scents? Burning a relaxing or sedating oils during breakfast time is not usually a good idea.

A citrus oil is fresh and clean and can help to lift feelings of lethargy and depression and get your family ready to face the day.

When winding down for bedtime, it is obviously better to use the more calming oils such as Lavender, Chamomile and Sandalwood.

When your kids are studying, help them to focus by burning oils like Rosemary and Peppermint.

When the kids are out and it is mom and dad's date night, it is time to pull out the more sensual oils like Ylang Ylang oil.

## Use Oils to Keep Everyone Healthy

You can also help to keep your family healthy by burning essential oils like Tea Tree, Eucalyptus and Lavender every day. These oils will help to clear out the germs in the air and will also help to improve the immunity of everyone in the house.

This can help to prevent the entire family getting sick.

## Use Blending as a Bonding Opportunity

Teens and tweens are likely to show some interests in the therapeutic properties of essential oils or, at the very least, are bound to enjoy blending their own perfumes and colognes.

Take the time to teach them what you have learned and you will have a valuable bonding opportunity.

Essential oils can do so much to keep you and your family healthy, happy and in good shape - they deserve a second look.

# Chapter 17: More Essential Oils

## Oils That you Might Want to Add to Your Kit

As you progress in your journey learning about the different properties of essential oils and how to use these to create natural health and beauty treatments, I am sure that you will want to increase your collection of oils. The following oils are nice to have but not entirely essential. Still, it could benefit you to get them.

### Tea Tree

Tea Tree is seldom chosen for its scent - it is medicinal and quite overpowering and I do not like it at all. That said, I do keep some on hand for small cuts, grazes or mild bacterial skin infections and also for fungal infections like ringworm. Tea Tree is one of the oils with the strongest anti-bacterial action and has the further distinction of being able to be applied neat.

My son used to battle with acne and would spot treat particularly angry looking spots with a blend of Lavender and Tea Tree oil - both applied neat. If dabbed onto inflamed, infected pustules, this helps to reduce swelling and redness and also fight the bacteria in the pimple.

Tea tree makes a great flea fighter and is very good to get rid of parasites and ringworm. The main reason that I use it despite not liking it is that there is no need to go to the trouble of diluting it when I have a small cut or infected piece of skin.

# Benzoin

You may find that Benzoin is one of those oils that is a little more difficult to fin a spot for in a blend but then again, even used on its own, its permeating vanilla scent is often enough to lift the spirits.

It can help ease a tight chest and is very valuable in the treatment of depression and stress. Blend equal parts Benzoin oil, Rose oil and Jasmine oil for a truly heavenly blend that smells wonderful and that will lift your spirits in no time flat.

This is a very sluggish liquid as it is derived from a resin and so I find that it is better used in a diffuser. A drop or so is all that is needed - it has a very rich aroma. Mixed with 2 drops each of Cedar Wood oil and Neroli oil an diffuser and you have the perfect blend to use when feeling overworked and under pressure.

# Jasmine

Jasmine absolute is rather expensive and, to be honest, out of most people's price ranges. That is not to say that you can never use it - Jasmine blends are available on the market and some of these are actually pretty good.

If you want to add Jasmine oil, stick to only a well-known, quality brand. You will pay extra but this is one of the most useful oils when it comes to creating feeling of content and in beating back depression.

Jasmine oil also has wonderful curative properties for the skin and will blend with almost all other essential oils. It can also help ease a hoarse throat.

Jasmine is a floral note and is quite penetrating so start with lower concentrations.

If you want to make floral perfumes or perfumes with a hint of the Orient, Jasmine is an oil that you must get. It helps to round off the more severe notes and to harmonize the blend overall.

## Rose

As with Jasmine absolute, pure Rose Otto is rather expensive and out of the range of most people. Again, there is no need to go without it though - choose a blend from a well-know, quality brand.

Rose is a wonderful base note  to use for a perfume and should always be included when trying to find the perfect blend of oils. Rose and Jasmine oil together are truly lovely. For a perfume that is out of this world, mix equal quantities of Rose oil, Jasmine oil, Ylang Ylang oil, Neroli oil and Sandalwood oil.

Rose is a wonderful anti-aging oil and can be used to soothe a wide range of skin ailments. It is particularly beneficial for irritated or burned skin and promotes the regeneration of tissue. It can help to minimize the looks of fine lines and thread veins.

And, as if all that was not enough, the oil is deeply relaxing and restorative and a valuable ally in the fight against depression.

## Basil

Basil is one of those oils that is not absolutely essential but it is a good oil to have on hand if you have teens that need to study for exams or if you yourself need to study or focus.

Mixing it with Bergamot and Lime can help tone down the scent a little. Mixing it with Citronella will mean that insects will give that area a wide berth.

It is not safe to use during pregnancy and may irritate the skin so care does need to be taken when using the oil. I use it in a diffuser as far as possible.

Diffused it is a good remedy for respiratory tract infections, colds, the flu and other infectious illnesses and it can clear out a brain fog quite fast. It is a good treatment for stress, anxiety, depression and fatigue.

Blended in low concentrations it is good for treating stomach upsets and menstrual cramping. It can help to relieve the pain associated with gout and also sore muscles and joints.

## Bergamot

Bergamot is quite a useful oil to have - it has strong anti-bacterial properties and is also an effective fungus fighter. It is good for treating vaginal discharge, cystitis, acne, boils, cold sores, eczema, insect repellent and insect bites, oily complexion, psoriasis, scabies, spots, varicose ulcers, wounds.

It can help get rid of bad breath and relieve infections of the mouth and tonsils.

It is also a valuable addition to the diffuser when colds and the flu strike.

It is a good oil to use to counter depression and to also combat sleeplessness caused by depression.

# Chapter 18: Cheat Sheet of Essential Oils' Benefits

## Your Two-Second Guide to Choosing the Right Oil

**Antiseptics** to treat cuts, insect bites, spots, etc. include Thyme oil, Sage oil, Eucalyptus oil, Tea Tree oil, Clove oil, Lavender oil and Lemon oil.

**Anti-inflammatory** oils to treat eczema, infected wounds, bumps, bruises, etc. include Chamomile oil, Lavender oil and Yarrow oil.

**Fungicidal** oils to treat athletes foot, candida, ringworm, etc. include Lavender, Tea Tree oil, Myrrh oil, Patchouli oil and Sweet Marjoram oil.

**Insect repellents and parasiticides** to get rid of lice, fleas, scabies, ticks, mosquitoes, ants, moths, etc. include Lavender oil, Garlic oil, Geranium oil, Citronella oil, Eucalyptus oil, Clove oil, Camphor oil and Cedar Wood oil.

**Hypotensives** to treat high blood pressure, palpitations, stress, etc. include Sweet Marjoram oil, Ylang Ylang oil, Lavender oil and Lemon oil.

**Hypertensives** to treat poor circulation, chilblains, listlessness, etc, include Rosemary oil, Lavender oil, Eucalyptus oil, Peppermint oil, Thyme oil.

**Rubefacients** to treat rheumatism of the joints, muscular stiffness, sciatica, lumbago, etc. include Black Pepper oil, Juniper oil, Rosemary, Camphor, Sweet Marjoram.

**Depurative or anti-toxic agents** to treat arthritis, gout, congestion, skin eruptions, etc. include Juniper oil, Lemon oil, Fennel oil and Lovage oil.

**Lymphatic stimulants** for cellulitis, obesity, water retention, etc. include Grapefruit oil, Lime oi, Fennel Oil, Lemon oil, Mandarin oil and White Birch oil.

**Circulatory tonics and astringents** for swellings, inflammations, varicose veins, etc. include Cypress oil, Yarrow oil, Lemon oil.

**Expectorants** for catarrh, sinusitis, coughs, bronchitis, etc. include Eucalyptus oil, Pine oil, Thyme oil, Myrrh oil, Sandalwood oil and Fennel oil.

**Antispasmodics** for colic, asthma, dry cough, whooping cough, etc. include Hyssop oil, Cypress oil, Cedar Wood, Bergamot, Chamomile and Cajeput.

**Balsamic agents** for colds, chills, congestion, etc. include Benzoin oil, Frankincense oil, Tolu Balsam oil, Peru Balsam oil, and Myrrh oil.

**Antiseptics** for 'flu, colds, sore throat, tonsillitis, gingivitis, etc. include Thyme oil, Sage oil, Eucalyptus oil, Hyssop oil, Pine oil, Cajeput oil, Tea Tree oil and Borneol oil.

**Antispasmodics** for spasm, pain, indigestion, etc. include Chamomile oil, Caraway oil, Fennel oil, Orange oil, Peppermint, Lemon Balm, Aniseed, Cinnamon.

**Carminatives and stomachics** for flatulent dyspepsia, aerophagia, nausea, etc. include Angelica oil, Basil oil, Fennel oil, Chamomile oil, Peppermint oil and Mandarin oil.

**Cholagogues** for increasing the flow of bile and stimulating the gall bladder include Caraway oil, Lavender oil, Peppermint Oil and Borneol oil.

**Hepatics** for liver congestion, jaundice, etc. include Lemon oil, Lime oil, Rosemary oil, Peppermint oil.

**Aperitifs** for loss of appetite, anorexia, etc, include Aniseed oil, Angelica oil, Orange oil, Ginger oil, Garlic oil.

**Antispasmodics** for menstrual cramp (dysmenorrhoea), labour pains, etc. include Sweet Marjoram oil, Chamomile oil, Clary Sage oil, Jasmine oil and Lavender oil.

**Emmenagogues** for scanty periods, lack of periods (amenorrhoea), etc. include Chamomile oil, Fennel oil, Hyssop oil, Juniper oil, Sweet Marjoram and Peppermint.

**Uterine tonics and regulators** for pregnancy, excess menstruation (menorrhagia), PMT, etc. include Clary Sage oil, Jasmine oil, Rose oil, Myrrh oil, Frankincense oil and Melissa oil.

**Antiseptic and bactericidal agents** for leucorrhoea, vaginal pruritis, thrush, etc. include Bergamot oil, Chamomile oil, Myrrh oil, Rose oil and Tea Tree oil.

**Anaphrodisiacs** for reducing sexual desire include Sweet Marjoram oil and Camphor oil.

**Adrenal stimulants** for anxiety, stress-related conditions, etc. include Basil oil, Geranium oil, Rosemary oil, Borneol oil, Sage oil, Pine oil and Savory oil.

**Urinary antiseptics** for cystitis, urethritis, etc. include Bergamot oil, Chamomile oil, Tea Tree oil and Sandalwood oil.

**Bactericidal and antiviral agents (prophylactics)** for protection against colds, the 'flu, etc include Tea Tree Oil, Cajeput oil, Niaouli oil, Basil oil, Lavender oil, Eucalyptus oil, Bergamot oil, Camphor oil, Clove oil, Rosemary oil.

**Febrifuge agents** for reducing fever and temperature, etc. include Angelica oil, Basil oil, Peppermint oil, Thyme oil, Sage oil, Lemon oil, Eucalyptus oil and Tea Tree oil.

**Sudorifics and diaphoretics** for promoting sweating, eliminating toxins, etc. include Rosemary oil, Thyme oil, Hyssop oil and Chamomile oil.

# Chapter 19: Cheat Sheet of Aromatherapy Blends

## Your Two-Second Guide to Which Oils Blend Well With One Another

I find that I work with the same four or five oils over and over again. Buying oils that blend well together makes perfect financial sense. It is important to start with a two oil blend. You can then select a third to round it off. Let's take the first entry below, Basil. Maybe you want to make a skin cleanser for oily skin so you choose Lemongrass, all good so far. You seen in the list with Basil is Geranium so you add that in as well and that is where it all goes wrong. Both Lemongrass and Geranium are a good match for basil but they are not a good match for each other.

Each oil in your blend should ideally blend with at least one of the other oils as well.

Here is your cheat sheet so that you can see which oil blends with the others easily:

**Basil:** Bergamot oil, Black Pepper oil, Clary Sage oil, Geranium oil, Hyssop oil, Lavender oil, Lemongrass oil, Marjoram oil, Melissa oil, Neroli oil and Sandalwood oil.

**Benzoin:** Bergamot oil, Cypress oil, Eucalyptus oil, Frankincense oil, Juniper oil, Lavender oil, Lemon oil, Myrrh oil, Orange oil, Petitgrain oil, Rose oil and Sandalwood oil.

**Bergamot:** Basil oil, Bergamot oil, Chamomile oil, Cypress oil, Eucalyptus oil, Geranium oil, Juniper oil, Jasmine oil, Lavender oil, Lemon oil, Sweet Marjoram oil, Neroli oil, Palmarosa oil, Patchouli oil and Ylang Ylang oil.

**Black Pepper:** Basil oil, Benzoin oil, Cypress oil, Frankincense oil, Geranium oil, Grapefruit oil, Lemon oil, Palmarosa oil, Rosemary oil, Sandalwood oil and Ylang Ylang oil.

**Cedar Wood:** Benzoin oil, Bergamot oil, Cinnamon oil, Cypress oil, Frankincense oil, Jasmine oil, Lavender oil, Lemon oil, Neroli oil, Rose oil and Rosemary oil.

**Chamomile:** Benzoin oil, Bergamot oil, Geranium oil, Juniper oil, Jasmine oil, Lavender oil, Lemon oil, Sweet Marjoram oil, Neroli oil, Palmarosa oil, Patchouli and Ylang Ylang oil.

**Cinnamon:** Benzoin oil, Clove oil, Frankincense oil, Ginger oil, Grapefruit oil, Lavender oil, Orange oil, Pine oil, Rosemary oi and Thyme oil.

**Clary Sage:** Basil oil, Bergamot oil, Cedar Wood oil, Cypress oil, Frankincense oil, Geranium oil, Grapefruit oil, Juniper oil, Jasmine oil, Lavender oil, and Sandalwood.

**Clove:** Basil oil, Benzoin oil, Black Pepper oil, Cinnamon oil, Grapefruit oil, Lemon oil, Nutmeg oil, Orange oil, Peppermint oil and Rosemary oil.

**Coriander:** Bergamot oil, Black Pepper oil, Cinnamon, Cypress oil and Geranium oil.

**Cypress:** Benzoin oil, Bergamot oil, Coriander oil, Juniper oil, Lavender oil, Lemon oil, Orange oil, Pine oil, Rosemary oil and Sandalwood oil.

**Eucalyptus:** Benzoin oil, Bergamot oil, Coriander oil, Juniper oil, Lavender oil, Lemon oil, Lemongrass oil, Melissa oil, Pine oil and Thyme oil.

**Fennel:** Basil oil, Geranium oil, Lavender oil, Lemon oil, Rose oil, Rosemary oil and Sandalwood oil.

**Frankincense:** Benzoin oil, Black Pepper oil, Geranium oil, Grapefruit oil, Lavender oil, Orange oil, Melissa oil, Patchouli oil, Pine oil and Sandalwood oil.

**Geranium:** Basil oil, Bergamot oil, Cedar Wood oil, Clary Sage oil, Grapefruit oil, Jasmine oil, Lavender oil, Lime oil, Neroli oil, Orange oil, Petitgrain oil, Rose, Rosemary and Sandalwood.

**Ginger:** All spice oils, Eucalyptus oil, Frankincense oil, Geranium oil, Lemon oil, Lime oil, Orange oil, Rosemary oil and Spearmint oil.

**Grapefruit:** Basil oil, Bergamot oil. Cedar Wood oil, Chamomile oil, Frankincense oil, Geranium oil, Jasmine oil, Lavender oil, Rosewood oil, Rose oil and Ylang Ylang oil.

**Hyssop:** Basil oil, Fennel oil, Lavender oil, Melissa oil, Orange oil, Rosemary oil and

Mandarin oil.

**Jasmine:** Blends with practically all other blends but particularly well with Bergamot oil, Frankincense oil, Geranium oil, Orange oil, Mandarin oil, Melissa oil, Neroli oil, Palmarosa oil, Rose oil, Rosewood and Sandalwood.

**Juniper:** Benzoin oil, Bergamot oil, Cypress oil, Frankincense oil, Geranium oil, Grapefruit oil, Orange oil, Lemon Grass oil, Lime oil, Melissa oil, Rosemary oil and Sandalwood oil.

**Lavender:** Lavender oil will blend with any other but is particularly good with the following oils - Basil oil, Benzoin oil, Bergamot oil, Chamomile oil, Clary Sage oil, Geranium oil, Jasmine oil, Lemon oil Lemongrass oil, Mandarin oil, Nutmeg oil, Orange oil, Patchouli oil, Pine oil, Rosemary oil and Thyme oil.

**Lemon:** Benzoin oil, Bergamot oil, Chamomile oil, Eucalyptus oil, Fennel oil, Frankincense oil, Ginger oil, Juniper oil, Lavender oil, Neroli oil, Rose oil, Sandalwood oil, Ylang Ylang oil.

**Lemon Grass:** Basil oil, Cedar Wood oil, Coriander oil, Geranium oil, Jasmine oil, Lavender oil, Neroli oil, Palmarosa oil, Rosemary oil, Tea Tree oil.

**Lime:** Bergamot oil, Geranium oil, Lavender oil, Neroli oil, Nutmeg oil, Palmarosa oil, Rose oil, Ylang Ylang oil.

**Mandarin:** Basil oil, Bergamot oil, Black Pepper oil, Coriander oil, Chamomile oil, Grapefruit oil, Lavender oil,Lemon oil, Lime oil, Sweet Marjoram oil, Neroli oil, Palmrosa oil, Petitgrain oil, Rose oil.

**Sweet Marjoram:** Basil oil, Bergamot oil, Cedar Wood oil, Chamomile oil, Cypress, Lavender oil, Mandarin oil, Orange oil, Neroli oil, Nutmeg oil,  Rosemary oil, Rosewood oil, Ylang Ylang oil.

**Melissa:** Basil oil, Chamomile oil, Frankincense oil, Geranium oil, Ginger oil, Jasmine oil, Lavender oil, Marjoram oil, Neroli oil, Rose oil, Rosemary oil, Ylang Ylang oil.

**Myrrh:** Benzoin oil, Clove oil, Chamomile oil, Frankincense oil, Lavender oil, Patchouli oil and Sandalwood oil.

**Neroli:** Basil oil, Benzoin oil, Bergamot oil, Coriander oil, Geranium oil, Jasmine oil, Lavender oil, Lemon oil, Lime oil, Orange oil, Palmarosa oil, Petitgrain oil, Rose oil, , Rosemary oil, Sandalwood oil, Ylang Ylang oil.

**Lemon:** Benzoin oil, Bergamot oil, Chamomile oil, Eucalyptus oil, Fennel oil, Frankincense oil, Ginger oil, Juniper oil, Lavender oil, Neroli oil, Rose oil, Sandalwood oil, Ylang Ylang oil.

**Niaouli:** Coriander oil, Fennel oil, Juniper oil, Lavender oil, Lemon oil, Lime oil, Orange oil, Pine oil, Peppermint oil, Rosemary oil.

**Nutmeg:** All other spice oils. All citrus oils. Cypress oil, Frankincense oil, Patchouli oil, Rosemary oil and Tea Tree oil.

**Orange:** Benzoin oil, Cinnamon oil, Coriander oil, Clove oil, Cypress oil, Frankincense oil, Geranium oil, Jasmine oil, Juniper oil, Lavender oil, Neroli oil, Nutmeg, Petitgrain, Rose oil, Rosewood oil and Sandalwood oil.

**Palmarosa:** Bergamot oil, Citronella oil, Geranium oil, Jasmine oil, Lavender oil, Lime oil, Melissa oil, Orange oil, Petitgrain oil, Rose oil, Rosewood oil, Sandalwood oil and Ylang Ylang oil.

**Patchouli:** Bergamot oil, Black Pepper oil, Clary Sage oil, Frankincense oil, Ginger oil, Lavender oil, Lemongrass oil, Myrrh, Neroli oil, Pine oil, Rose oil, Rosewood oil and Sandalwood oil.

**Peppermint:** Benzoin oil, Cedar Wood oil, Cypress oil, Lavender oil, Mandarin oil, Sweet Marjoram oil, Niaouli oil, Pine oil and Rosemary oil.

**Petitgrain:** Benzoin oil, Bergamot oil, Cedar Wood oil, Geranium oil, Lavender oil, Melissa oil, Neroli oil, Orange oil, Palmarosa oil, Rosemary oil, Rosewood oil and Sandalwood oil.

**Pine:** Cedar Wood oil, Cinnamon Oil, Clove oil, Cypress oil, Eucalyptus oil, Lavender oil, Niaouli oil, Rosemary oil, Thyme oil and Tea Tree oil.

**Rose:** This is another of the oils that will blend with just about any other oil. Rose oil blends best with the following oils - Benzoin oil, Bergamot oil, Chamomile oil, Clary Sage oil, Geranium oil, Jasmine oil, Lavender oil, Neroli oil, Orange oil, Palmarosa oil, Patchouli oil and Sandalwood oil.

**Rosemary:** Basil oil, Cedar Wood oil, Frankincense oil, Geranium oil, Ginger oil, Grapefruit oil, Lavender oil, Lemongrass oil, Lime oil, Mandarin oil, Melissa oil, Orange oil and Peppermint oil.

**Rosewood:** Cedar Wood oil, Coriander oil, Frankincense, Geranium, Pamlarosa, Patchouli, Petitgrain, Rose, Rosemary, Sandalwood, Vetiver.

**Sandalwood:** Basil oil, Benzoin oil, Black Pepper oil, Cypress oil, Frankincense oil, Geranium oil, Jasmine oil, Lavender oil, Lemon oil, Myrrh oil, Neroli oil, Palmarosa oil, Rose oil, Vetiver oil and Ylang Ylang oil.

**Thyme:** Bergamot oil, Cedar Wood oil, Chamomile oil, Juniper oil, Lavender oil, Lemon oil, Niaouli oil, Mandarin oil, Melissa oil, Rosemary oil and Tea Tree oil.

**Vetiver:** Benzoin oil, Frankincense oil, Geranium oil, Grapefruit oil, Jasmine oil, Lavender oil, Patchouli oil, Rose oil, Rosewood oil,Sandalwood oil and Ylang Ylang oil.

**Ylang Ylang:** Bergamot oil, Grapefruit oil, Jasmine oil, Lavender oil, Lemon oil, Melissa oil, Neroli oil, Orange oil, Patchouli oil, Rose oil,  Rosewood oil,Sandalwood oil, and Vetiver oil.

This is a basic cheat sheet and is a good place to start. You may find that some oils that you would expect to be listed are not. On this cheat sheet, the very best oils for blending with one another were chosen so that there is little room for error for the person just setting out.

As you get more experienced, I do urge you to start making up your own blends, even if they do not seem to be good according to the above-mentioned list. As long as the oils are compatible with one another, you will get a really good and useful blend that is better overall than it is in separate parts.

According to the list above, Sandalwood and Bergamot, for example, are not ideal blends. In reality, I quite like that particular blend and find it useful when I am feeling under pressure.

As I mentioned before, blending oils is largely an art and based very much upon personal preferences. Follow the guidelines until you are confident to try making your own rules and you could have a winning formula on your hands. Use small quantities of oils if you are not sure how the blend will turn out and then not much time or money is wasted, leaving you free to work on improving on the ideas that didn't quite go the distance in terms of efficacy or scent.

# Chapter 20: Cheat Sheet of Application Tips

## Your Two-Second Guide to Using Aromatherapy Oils

This is a very rough guide to help you choose oils that are good for helping with conditions that you or a family member may suffer from.

I advise choosing a few different oils from the relevant categories and then checking what oils can be blended together successfully. Choose a blend from that list, making sure that the symptoms that you want to treat are covered and that the blend will appeal to you or to the person that you are making it for.

Check the contraindications for the chosen oils before adding them to your blend.

## Skin Care

**Acne:** Bergamot, camphor (white), cananga, cedar wood, chamomile, clove bud, galbanum, geranium, grapefruit, helichrysum, juniper, lavandin, lavender, lemon, lemongrass, lime, linaloe, litsea cubeba, mandarin, mint, myrtle, niaouli, palmarosa, patchouli, petitgrain, rosemary, rosewood, clary sage, sandalwood, tea tree, thyme, vetiver, violet, yarrow and ylang ylang oils.

**Allergies** : Lemon balm, chamomile, helichrysum, true lavender oils.

**Athlete's Foot:** Clove bud, eucalyptus, lavender (true & spike), lemon, lemongrass, myrrh, patchouli, tea tree oil.

**Baldness & Hair Care:** West Indian bay, white birch, cedar wood (Atlas, Texas & Virginian), chamomile (German & Roman), grapefruit, juniper, patchouli, rosemary, sage (clary & Spanish), yarrow and ylang ylang oils.

**Boils, abscesses & blisters:** Bergamot, chamomile (German & Roman), eucalyptus blue gum, galbanum, helichrysum, lavandin, lavender (spike & true), lemon, mastic, niaouli, clary sage, tea tree, thyme and turpentine oils.

**Bruises:** Arnica (cream), borneol, clove bud, fennel, geranium, hyssop, sweet marjoram, lavender and thyme oils.

**Burns:** Canadian balsam, chamomile (German & Roman), clove bud, eucalyptus blue gum, geranium, helichrysum, lavandin, lavender (spike & true), marigold, niaouli, tea tree and yarrow oils.

**Chapped & cracked skin:** Peru balsam, Tolu balsam, benzoin, myrrh, patchouli and sandalwood oils.

**Chilblains:** Chamomile (German & Roman), lemon, lime, sweet marjoram and black pepper oils.

**Cold sores/herpes:** Bergamot, eucalyptus blue gum, lemon and tea tree oils.

**Congested & dull skin:** Angelica, white birch, sweet fennel, geranium, grapefruit, lavandin, lavender (spike & true), lemon, lime, mandarin, mint (peppermint & spearmint), myrtle, niaouli, orange (bitter & sweet), palmarosa, rose (cabbage & damask), rosemary, rosewood and ylang ylang oils.

**Cuts/sores:** Canadian balsam, benzoin, borneol, cabreuva, cade, chamomile (German & Roman), clove bud, elemi, eucalyptus (blue gum, lemon & peppermint), galbanum, geranium, helichrysum, hyssop, lavandin, lavender (spike & true), lemon, lime, linaloe, marigold, mastic, myrrh, niaouli, Scotch pine, Spanish sage, Levant styrax, tea tree, thyme, turpentine, vetiver and yarrow oils.

**Dandruff:** West Indian bay, cade, cedarwood (Atlas, Texas & Virginian), eucalyptus, spike lavender, lemon, patchouli, rosemary, sage (clary & Spanish) and tea tree oils.

**Dermatitis:** White birch, cade, cananga, carrot seed, cedarwood (Atlas, Texas & Virginian), chamomile (German & Roman), geranium, helichrysum, hops, hyssop, juniper, true lavender, linaloe, litsea cubeba, mint (peppermint & spearmint), palmarosa, patchouli, rosemary, sage (clary & Spanish) and thyme oils.

**Dry & sensitive skin:** Peru balsam, Tolu balsam, cassie, chamomile (German & Roman), frankincense, jasmine, lavandin, lavender (spike & true), rosewood, sandalwood and violet oils.

**Eczema:** Lemon balm, Peru balsam, Tolu balsam, bergamot, white birch, cade, carrot seed, cedarwood (Atlas, Texas & Virginian), chamomile (German & Roman), geranium, helichrysum, hyssop, juniper, lavandin, lavender (spike & true), marigold, myrrh, patchouli, rose (cabbage & damask), rosemary, Spanish sage, thyme, violet and yarrow oils.

**Excessive perspiration:** Citronella, cypress, lemongrass, litsea cubeba, petitgrain, Scotch pine and Spanish sage oils.

**Greasy or oily skin/scalp:** West Indian bay, bergamot, cajeput, camphor (white), cananga, carrot seed, citronella, cypress, sweet fennel, geranium, jasmine, juniper, lavender, lemon, lemongrass, litsea cubeba, mandarin, marigold, mimosa, myrtle, niaouli, palmarosa, patchouli, petitgrain, rosemary, rosewood, sandalwood, clary sage, tea tree, thyme, vetiver and ylang ylang oils.

**Haemorrhoids/piles:** Canadian balsam, Copaiba balsam, coriander, cubebs, cypress, geranium, juniper, myrrh, myrtle, parsley and yarrow oils.

**Insect bites:** Lemon balm, French basil, bergamot, cajeput, cananga, chamomile (German & Roman), cinnamon leaf, eucalyptus blue gum, lavandin, lavender (spike & true), lemon, marigold, niaouli, tea tree, thyme and ylang ylang oils.

**Insect repellent:** Lemon balm, French basil, bergamot, borneol, camphor (white), Virginian cedarwood, citronella, clove bud, cypress, eucalyptus (blue gum & lemon), geranium, lavender, lemongrass, litsea cubeba, mastic, patchouli, rosemary, turpentine.

**Irritated & inflamed skin:** Angelica, benzoin, camphor (white), Atlas cedar wood, chamomile (German & Roman), elemi, helichrysum, hyssop, jasmine, lavandin, true lavender, marigold, myrrh, patchouli, rose (cabbage & damask), clary sage, spikenard, tea tree, yarrow.

**Lice:** Cinnamon leaf, eucalyptus blue gum, galbanum, geranium, lavandin, spike lavender, parsley, Scotch pine, rosemary, thyme, turpentine.

**Mouth & gum infections/ulcers:** Bergamot, cinnamon leaf, cypress, sweet fennel, lemon, mastic, myrrh, orange (bitter & sweet), sage (clary & Spanish), thyme.

**Psoriasis:** Angelica, bergamot, white birch, carrot seed, chamomile (German & Roman), true lavender.

**Rashes:** Peru balsam, Tolu balsam, carrot seed, chamomile (German & Roman), hops, true lavender, marigold, sandalwood, spikenard, tea tree, yarrow.

**Ringworm:** Geranium, spike lavender, mastic, mint (peppermint & spearmint), myrrh, Levant styrax, tea tree, turpentine.

**Scabies:** Tolu balsam, bergamot, cinnamon leaf, lavandin, lavender (spike & true), lemongrass, mastic, mint (peppermint & spearmint), Scotch pine, rosemary, Levant styrax, thyme, turpentine.

**Scars & stretch marks:** Cabreuva, elemi, frankincense, galbanum, true lavender, mandarin, orange blossom, palmarosa, patchouli, rosewood, sandalwood, spikenard, violet, yarrow.

**Slack tissue:** Geranium, grapefruit, juniper, lemongrass, lime, mandarin, sweet marjoram, orange blossom, black pepper, petitgrain, rosemary, yarrow.

**Spots:** Bergamot, cade, cajeput, camphor (white), eucalyptus (lemon), helichrysum, lavandin, lavender (spike & true), lemon, lime, litsea cubeba, mandarin, niaouli, tea tree.

**Ticks:** Sweet marjoram.

**Toothache & teething pain:** Chamomile (German & Roman), clove bud, mastic, mint (peppermint & spearmint), myrrh.

**Varicose veins:** Cypress, lemon, lime, orange blossom, yarrow.

**Veruccae:** Tagetes, tea tree.

**Warts & corns:** Cinnamon leaf, lemon, lime, tagetes, tea tree.

**Wounds:** Canadian balsam, Peru balsam, Tolu balsam, bergamot, cabreuva, chamomile (German & Roman), clove bud, cypress, elemi, eucalyptus (blue gum & lemon), frankincense, galbanum, geranium, helichrysum, hyssop, juniper, lavandin, lavender (spike & true), linaloe, marigold, mastic, myrrh, niaouli, patchouli, rosewood, Levant styrax, tea tree, turpentine, vetiver, yarrow.

**Wrinkles & mature skin:** Carrot seed, elemi, sweet fennel, frankincense, galbanum, geranium, jasmine, labdanum, true lavender, mandarin, mimosa, myrrh, orange blossom, palmarosa, patchouli, rose (cabbage & damask), rosewood, clary sage, sandalwood, spikenard, ylang ylang.

## Circulation, Muscles and Joints:

**Accumulation of toxins:** Angelica, white birch, carrot seed, celery seed, coriander, cumin, sweet fennel, grapefruit, juniper, lovage, parsley.

**Aches and pains:** Ambrette, star anise, aniseed, French basil, West Indian bay, cajeput, calamintha, camphor (white), chamomile (German & Roman), coriander, eucalyptus (blue gum & peppermint), silver fir, galbanum, ginger, helichrysum, lavandin, lavender (spike & true), lemongrass, sweet marjoram, mastic, mint (peppermint & spearmint), niaouli, nutmeg, black pepper, pine (longleaf & Scotch), rosemary, sage (clary & Spanish), hemlock spruce, thyme, turmeric, turpentine, vetiver.

**Arthritis:** Allspice, angelica, benzoin, white birch, cajeput, camphor (white), carrot seed, cedar wood (Atlas, Texas & Virginian), celery seed, chamomile (German & Roman), clove bud, coriander, eucalyptus (blue gum & peppermint), silver fir, ginger, guaiacwood, juniper, lemon, sweet marjoram, mastic, myrrh, nutmeg, parsley, black pepper, pine (longleaf & Scotch), rosemary, Spanish sage, thyme, tumeric, turpentine, vetiver, yarrow.

**Cellulitis:** White birch, cypress, sweet fennel, geranium, grapefruit, juniper, lemon, parsley, rosemary, thyme.

**Debility/poor muscle tone:** Allspice, ambrette, borneol, ginger, grapefruit, sweet marjoram, black pepper, pine (longleaf & Scotch), rosemary, Spanish sage.

**Gout:** Angelica, French basil, benzoin, carrot seed, celery seed, coriander, guaiacwood, juniper, lovage, mastic, pine (longleaf & Scotch), rosemary, thyme, turpentine.

**High blood pressure & hypertension:** Lemon balm, cananga, garlic, true lavender, lemon, sweet marjoram, clary sage, yarrow, ylang ylang.

**Muscular cramp & stiffness:** Allspice, ambrette, coriander, cypress, grapefruit, jasmine, lavandin, lavender (spike & true), sweet marjoram, black pepper, pine (longleaf & Scotch), rosemary, thyme, vetiver.

**Obesity:** White birch, sweet fennel, juniper, lemon, mandarin, orange (bitter & sweet).

**Oedema & water retention:** Angelica, white birch, carrot seed, cypress, sweet fennel, geranium, grapefruit, juniper, lovage, mandarin, orange (bitter &c sweet), rosemary, Spanish sage.

**Palpitations:** Orange (bitter & sweet), orange blossom, rose (cabbage & damask), ylang ylang.

**Poor circulation & low blood pressure:** Ambrette, Peru balsam, West Indian bay, benzoin, white birch, borneol, cinnamon leaf, coriander, cumin, cypress, eucalyptus blue gum, galbanum, geranium, ginger, lemon, lemongrass, lovage, niaouli, nutmeg, orange blossom, black pepper, pine (longleaf & Scotch), rose (cabbage & damask), rosemary, Spanish sage, hemlock spruce, thyme, violet.

**Rheumatism:** Allspice, angelica, star anise, aniseed, Peru balsam, French basil, West Indian bay, benzoin, white birch, borneol, cajeput, calamintha, camphor (white), carrot seed, cedar wood (Atlas, Texas & Virginian), celery seed, chamomile (German & Roman), cinnamon leaf, clove bud, coriander, cypress, eucalyptus (blue gum & peppermint), sweet fennel, silver fir, galbanum, ginger, helichrysum, juniper, lavandin, lavender (spike & true), lemon, lovage, sweet marjoram, mastic, niaouli, nutmeg, parsley, black pepper, pine (longleaf & Scotch), rosemary, Spanish sage, hemlock spruce, thyme, turmeric, turpentine, vetiver, violet, yarrow.

**Sprains & strains:** West Indian bay, borneol, camphor (white), chamomile (German & Roman), clove bud, eucalyptus (blue gum & peppermint), ginger, helichrysum, jasmine, lavandin, lavender (spike & true), sweet marjoram, black pepper, pine (longleaf & Scotch), rosemary, thyme, turmeric, vetiver.

# Respiratory System

**Asthma:** Asafetida, lemon balm, Canadian balsam, Peru balsam, benzoin, cajeput, clove bud, costus, cypress, elecampane, eucalyptus (blue gum, lemon & peppermint), frankincense, galbanum, helichrysum, hops, hyssop, lavandin, lavender (spike & true), lemon, lime, sweet marjoram, mint (peppermint & spearmint), myrrh, myrtle, niaouli, pine (longleaf & Scotch), rose (cabbage & damask), rosemary, sage (clary & Spanish), hemlock spruce, tea tree, thyme.

**Bronchitis:** Angelica, star anise, aniseed, asafetida, lemon balm, Canadian balsam, copaiba balsam, Peru balsam, Tolu balsam, French basil, benzoin, borneol, cajeput, camphor (white), caraway, cascarilla bark, cedar wood (Atlas, Texas & Virginian), clove bud, costus, cubebs, cypress, elecampane, elemi, eucalyptus (blue gum & peppermint), silver fir, frankincense, galbanum, helichrysum, hyssop, labdanum, lavandin, lavender (spike & true), lemon, sweet marjoram, mastic, mint (peppermint & spearmint), myrrh, myrtle, niaouli, orange (bitter & sweet), pine (longleaf & Scotch), rosemary, sandalwood, hemlock spruce, Levant styrax, tea tree, thyme, turpentine, violet.

**Catarrh:** Canadian balsam, Tolu balsam, cajeput, cedar wood (Atlas, Texas & Virginian), cubebs, elecampane, elemi, eucalyptus (blue gum & peppermint), frankincense, galbanum, ginger, hyssop, jasmine, lavandin, lavender (spike & true), lemon, lime, mastic, mint (peppermint & spearmint), myrrh, myrtle, niaouli, black pepper, pine (longleaf & Scotch), sandalwood, Levant styrax, tea tree, thyme, turpentine, violet.

**Chill**: Copaiba balsam, benzoin, cabreuva, calamintha, camphor (white), cinnamon leaf, ginger, grapefruit, orange (bitter & sweet), black pepper.

**Chronic coughs:** Melissa, Canadian balsam, costus, cubebs, cypress, elecampane, elemi, frankincense, galbanum, helichrysum, hops, hyssop, jasmine, mint (peppermint & spearmint), myrrh, myrtle, sandalwood, Levant styrax.

**Coughs:** Angelica, star anise, aniseed, copaiba balsam, Peru balsam, Tolu balsam, French basil , benzoin, borneol, cabreuva, cajeput, camphor (white), caraway, cascarilla bark, Atlas cedar wood, eucalyptus (blue gum & peppermint), silver fir, ginger, hyssop, labdanum, sweet marjoram, myrrh, niaouli, black pepper, pine (longleaf & Scotch), rose (cabbage & damask), rosemary, sage (clary & Spanish), hemlock spruce, tea tree.

**Croup:** Tolu balsam.

**Earache:** French basil, chamomile (German & Roman), lavender (spike & true).

**Halitosis/offensive breath:** Bergamot, cardomon, sweet fennel, lavandin, lavender (spike & true), mint (peppermint & spearmint), myrrh.

**Laryngitis/hoarseness:** Tolu balsam, benzoin, caraway, cubebs, lemon eucalyptus, frankincense, jasmine, lavandin, lavender (spike & true), myrrh, sage (clary & Spanish), sandalwood, thyme.

**Sinusitis:** French basil, cajeput, cubebs, eucalyptus blue gum, silver fir, ginger, labdanum, peppermint, niaouli, pine (longleaf & Scotch), tea tree.

**Sore throat & throat infections:** Canadian balsam, bergamot, cajeput, eucalyptus (blue gum, lemon & peppermint), geranium, ginger, hyssop, lavandin, lavender (spike & true), myrrh, myrtle, niaouli, pine (longleaf & Scotch), sage (clary & Spanish), sandalwood, tea tree, thyme, violet.

**Tonsillitis:** Bay laurel, bergamot, geranium, hyssop, myrtle, sage (clary & Spanish), thyme.

**Whooping cough:** Asafetida, helichrysum, hyssop, true lavender, mastic, niaouli, rosemary, sage (clary & Spanish), tea tree, turpentine.

# Digestive System

**Colic:** Star anise, aniseed, lemon balm, calamintha, caraway, cardomon, carrot seed, chamomile (German & Roman), clove bud, coriander, cumin, dill, sweet fennel, ginger, hyssop, lavandin, lavender (spike & true), sweet marjoram, mint (peppermint & spearmint), orange blossom, parsley, black pepper, rosemary, clary sage.

**Constipation & sluggish digestion:** Cinnamon leaf, cubebs, sweet fennel, lovage, sweet marjoram, nutmeg, orange (bitter & sweet), palmarosa, black pepper, tarragon, turmeric, yarrow.

**Cramp/gastric spasm:** Allspice, star anise, aniseed, caraway, cardamon, cinnamon leaf, coriander, costus, cumin, galbanum, ginger, lavandin, lavender (spike & true), lovage, mint (peppermint & spearmint), orange (bitter & sweet), orange blossom, black pepper, clary sage, tarragon, lemon verbena, yarrow.

**Griping pains:** Cardamon, dill, sweet fennel, parsley.

**Heartburn:** Cardamon, black pepper.

**Indigestion/flatulence:** Allspice, angelica, star anise, aniseed, lemon balm, French basil, bay laurel, calamintha, caraway, cardamon, carrot seed, cascarilla bark, celery seed, chamomile (German & Roman), cinnamon leaf, clove bud, coriander, costus, cubebs, cumin, dill, sweet fennel, galbanum, ginger, hops, hyssop, lavandin, lavender (spike & true), lemongrass, linden, litsea cubeba, lovage, mandarin, sweet marjoram, mint (peppermint & spearmint), myrrh, nutmeg, orange (bitter & sweet), orange blossom, parsley, black pepper, petitgrain, rosemary, clary sage, tarragon, thyme, valerian, lemon verbena, yarrow.

**Liver congestion:** Carrot seed, celery seed, helichrysum, linden, rose (cabbage & damask), rosemary, Spanish sage, turmeric, lemon verbena.

**Loss of appetite:** Bay laurel, bergamot, caraway, cardamon, ginger, myrrh, black pepper.

**Nausea/vomiting:** Allspice, lemon balm, French basil, cardamom, chamomile (German & Roman), clove bud, coriander, sweet fennel, ginger, lavandin, lavender (spike & true), mint (peppermint & spearmint), nutmeg, black pepper, rose (cabbage & damask), rosewood, sandalwood.

# Genito-Urinary and Endocrine Systems

**Amenorrhoea/lack of menstruation:** French basil, bay laurel, carrot seed, celery seed, cinnamon leaf, dill, sweet fennel, hops, hyssop, juniper, lovage, sweet marjoram, myrrh, parsley, rose (cabbage & damask), sage (clary & Spanish), tarragon, yarrow.

**Dysmenorrhoea/cramp, painful or difficult menstruation:** Lemon balm, French basil, carrot seed, chamomile (German & Roman), cypress, frankincense, hops, jasmine, juniper, lavandin, lavender (spike & true), lovage, sweet marjoram, rose (cabbage & damask), rosemary, sage (clary & Spanish), tarragon, yarrow.

**Cystitis:** Canadian balsam, copaiba balsam, bergamot, cedar wood (Atlas, Texas & Virginian), celery seed, chamomile (German & Roman), cubebs, eucalyptus blue gum, frankincense, juniper, lavandin, lavender (spike & true), lovage, mastic, niaouli, parsley, Scotch pine, sandalwood, tea tree, thyme, turpentine, yarrow.

**Frigidity:** Cassie, cinnamon leaf, jasmine, nutmeg, orange blossom, parsley, patchouli, black pepper, cabbage rose, rosewood, clary sage, sandalwood, ylang ylang.

**Lack of nursing milk:** Celery seed, dill, sweet fennel, hops.

**Labour pain & childbirth aid:** Cinnamon leaf, jasmine, true lavender, nutmeg, parsley, rose (cabbage & damask), clary sage.

**Leucorrhoea/white discharge from the vagina**: Bergamot, cedar wood (Atlas, Texas & Virginian), cinnamon leaf, cubebs, eucalyptus blue gum, frankincense, hyssop, lavandin, lavender (spike & true), sweet marjoram, mastic, myrrh, rosemary, clary sage, sandalwood, tea tree, turpentine.

**Menopausal problems:** Cypress, sweet fennel, geranium, jasmine, rose (cabbage & damask).

**Menorrhagia/excessive menstruation:** Chamomile (German & Roman), cypress, rose (cabbage & damask).

**Premenstrual tension /PMT:** Carrot seed, chamomile (German & Roman), geranium, true lavender, sweet marjoram, orange blossom, tarragon.

**Pruritis/itching:** Bergamot, Atlas cedar wood, juniper, lavender, myrrh, tea tree.

**Sexual over activity:** Hops, sweet marjoram.

**Thrush/candida:** Bergamot, geranium, myrrh, tea tree.

**Urethritis:** Bergamot, cubebs, mastic, tea tree, turpentine.

**Chickenpox:** Bergamot, chamomile (German & Roman), eucalyptus (blue gum & lemon), true lavender, tea tree.

**Colds/'flu:** Angelica, star anise, aniseed, copaiba balsam, Peru balsam, French basil, bay laurel, West Indian bay, bergamot, borneol, cabreuva, cajeput, camphor (white), caraway, cinnamon leaf, citronella, clove bud, coriander, eucalyptus (blue gum, lemon & peppermint), silver fir, frankincense, ginger, grapefruit, helichrysum, juniper, lemon, lime, sweet marjoram, mastic, mint (peppermint & spearmint), myrtle, niaouli, orange (bitter & sweet), pine (longleaf & Scotch), rosemary, rosewood, Spanish sage, hemlock spruce, tea tree, thyme, turpentine, yarrow.

**Fever:** French basil, bergamot, borneol, camphor (white), eucalyptus (blue gum, lemon & peppermint), silver fir, ginger, helichrysum, juniper, lemon, lemongrass, lime, mint (peppermint & spearmint), myrtle, niaouli, rosemary, rosewood, Spanish sage, hemlock spruce, tea tree, thyme, yarrow.

**Measles:** Bergamot, eucalyptus blue gum, lavender (spike & true), tea tree.

## Nervous System

**Anxiety:** Ambrette, lemon balm, French basil, bergamot, cananga, frankincense, hyssop, jasmine, juniper, true lavender, mimosa, orange blossom, hemlock spruce, Levant styrax, lemon verbena, ylang ylang.

**Depression:** Allspice, ambrette, lemon balm, Canadian balsam, French basil, bergamot, cassie, grapefruit, helichrysum, jasmine, true lavender, orange blossom, rose (cabbage & damask), clary sage, sandalwood, hemlock spruce, vetiver, ylang ylang.

**Headache:** Chamomile (German & Roman), citronella, cumin, eucalyptus (blue gum & peppermint), grapefruit, hops, lavandin, lavender (spike & true), lemongrass, linden, sweet marjoram, mint (peppermint & spearmint), rose (cabbage & damask), rosemary, rosewood, sage (clary & Spanish), thyme, violet.

**Insomnia:** Lemon balm, French basil, calamintha, chamomile (German & Roman), hops, true lavender, linden, mandarin, sweet marjoram, orange blossom, petitgrain, rose (cabbage & damask), sandalwood, thyme, valerian, lemon verbena, vetiver, violet, yarrow, ylang ylang.

**Migraine:** Angelica, lemon balm, French basil, chamomile (German & Roman), citronella, coriander, true lavender, linden, sweet marjoram, mint (peppermint & spearmint), clary sage, valerian, yarrow.

**Nervous exhaustion or fatigue/debility:** Allspice, angelica, asafetida, French basil, borneol, cardamon, cassie, cinnamon leaf, citronella, coriander, costus, cumin, elemi, eucalyptus (blue gum & peppermint), ginger, grapefruit, helichrysum, hyacinth, hyssop, jasmine, lavandin, spike lavender, lemongrass, mint (peppermint & spearmint), nutmeg, palmarosa, patchouli, petitgrain, Scotch pine, rosemary, sage (clary & Spanish), thyme, vetiver, violet, ylang ylang.

**Neuralgia/sciatica:** Allspice, West Indian bay, borneol, celery seed, chamomile (German & Roman), citronella, coriander, eucalyptus (blue gum & peppermint), geranium, helichrysum, hops, spike lavender, sweet marjoram, mastic, mint (peppermint & spearmint), nutmeg, pine (long leaf & Scotch), rosemary, turpentine.

**Nervous tension and stress:** Allspice, ambrette, angelica, asafetida, lemon balm, Canadian balsam, copaiba balsam, Peru balsam, French basil, benzoin, bergamot, borneol, calamintha, cananga, cardamon, cassie, cedar wood (Atlas, Texas & Virginian), chamomile (German & Roman) , cinnamon leaf, costus, cypress, elemi, frankincense, galbanum, geranium, helichrysum, hops, hyacinth, hyssop, jasmine, juniper, true lavender, lemongrass, linaloe, linden, mandarin, sweet marjoram, mimosa, mint (peppermint & spearmint), orange (bitter & sweet), orange blossom, palmarosa, patchouli, petitgrain, Scotch pine, rose (cabbage & damask), rosemary, rosewood, clary sage, sandalwood, hemlock spruce, thyme, valerian, lemon verbena, vetiver, violet, yarrow, ylang ylang.

**Shock:** Lemon balm, lavandin, lavender (spike & true), orange blossom.

**Vertigo:** Lemon balm, lavandin, lavender (spike & true), mint (peppermint & spearmint), violet.

# Conclusion

Thank you again for downloading this book!

I really hope that this book has taught you a lot and encouraged you to go out and explore the fascinating topic of aromatherapy.

I have been using essential oils for more than two decades now and I hardly ever need to go to the doctor. I never bother with an annual flu shot because I seldom get the flu.

Essential oils used on a regular basis can be as effective as commercial medications, treatments and cosmetic products. In fact, they are often more effective.

I hope that this book has taught you some valuable ways to help your own family on a daily basis and help you all to become happier, healthier, more vital and too ward off the effects of aging.

I know, I sound a bit like one of those old-time con artists selling a "miracle" cure-all and it may all seem a little too good to be true. The fact is though that while there is no one particular oil that can cover every eventuality, Lavender does come pretty close. As for efficacy of the oils - with over six thousands years in development, we can rest assured that essential oils are no fly-by-night remedy and that they deserve a place on your night stands.

Well, all that is left now is for you to go and make your own blends. Have a great time doing that - it is really fun.

Lastly, I would really appreciate it if you would let me know what you thought of this book by posting a review on Amazon.

Thank you so much and I wish you good blends!